Dr Alexander Logan

Get Me Into Medical School! S

Medical School Interviews

© Meddicle Publishing 2015

www.getmeintomedicalschool.com

Cover design by A Logan

Book design by A Logan

Character design by G Young

All rights reserved.

ISBN-13: 978-0993113826

ISBN-10: 0993113826

Get Me Into Medical School! Series

1. Should I Become A Doctor?

2. The Medical Schools Guide

3. Medical School Interviews

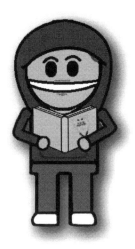

Download the Free App on the App Store

www.getmeintomedicalschool.com

Introduction

Welcome to the third book in our popular Get Me Into Medical School Series. By picking up this book we can assume that you are 100% certain that medicine is the career for you. Good decision. Being a doctor is a fantastic job with a multitude of possible career paths and a huge variety of patients, colleagues, specialties and diseases to discover.

This book was written entirely by medical school interviewers and recently successful candidates to give you all the inside information, tips and tricks required to not only do well at medical school interviews but to gain as many offers as possible and provide you with a choice of medical schools at which to study.

The book is divided into five simple chapters: chapter one covers how to write your personal statement, chapter two deals with overall interview technique and chapters three to five give you practise questions with comprehensive answers covering traditional, ethical and multiple mini interview (MMI) scenarios.

The best way to ensure success is to practise as much as possible.

Good luck. We'll see you at medical school.

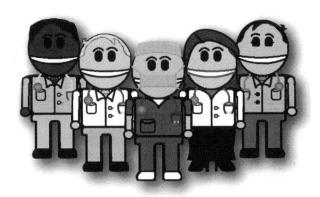

Chapter 1 The Personal Statement

Once you have chosen four medical schools to apply to the next step is to complete the UCAS form and write your personal statement. It is important to write the best personal statement that you can to ensure that you get called to interview.

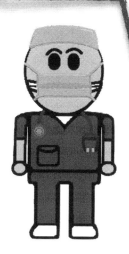

UCAS OVERVIEW

The Universities and Colleges Admissions Service (UCAS) organises all applications to medical courses in the UK including graduate entry and premedical courses.

The UCAS application system is only available online and it is important that you familiarise yourself with their website well ahead of the application deadline.

The UCAS website (www.UCAS.com) has lots of useful information ranging from application advice to specific information about each university. While the UCAS application is step three in your route to medical school (following getting top exam grades and medical admission tests and before the interview) it is worth looking through their website early to give you an idea of how to apply.

The UCAS application contains your personal details, exam results or predicted grades, school references and personal statement. It is the culmination of all the hard work you have put in through revision, work experience and extracurricular activities.

The process can be daunting and making your application stand out from all the others in the limited space provided can seem impossible. In this section we guide you through the application process and offer some top tips before looking in detail at how to write the best personal statement possible.

The Basics

Before looking at the application process in general it is important to know a few key facts.

Applications Open You may submit your UCAS application from mid-September. This gives you the entire summer to hone your personal statement and get it submitted as soon as the application system opens.

Application Deadline The deadline for medical school applications to be submitted is usually 15th October each year (check the UCAS website for the most up-to-date information). This is earlier than most other university courses but we advise getting the application in as soon as possible to maximise your chances of getting an interview.

Course Choices You can apply to six university courses through UCAS each year. For medicine you may only choose four courses and if you apply to Oxbridge you may choose Oxford or Cambridge not both. The remaining two spaces may be filled with alternative, non-medical courses if you want a back-up option.

UCAS Codes Medical courses for each university are coded using a UCAS code such as A100 for the standard undergraduate course and you will see this code on medical school admissions pages, prospectuses and the UCAS website.

Deferred Entry If you want to defer your entry to the following year to take a gap year there is a specific tick-box on the application form. Make sure that you check that the medical schools you are applying to accept deferred entry before ticking the box.

Application Fee UCAS charges £19 for your application. This is paid online during the application process.

Scoring UCAS passes on all the information within the application to your chosen four medical schools. Each medical school has an admissions department comprising of specialised staff and local doctors who then score the information within the application based on the specific medical school's guidelines.

Guide to the Application Form

The UCAS website offers easy to follow instructions and advice on how to complete the online application. Below is a summary of the key steps so you know what to expect.

Registration The registration process is quick, asking for your personal details and a valid email address. You will also choose a username and password and it is important that you keep these safe so that you can login to your application.

The Form The application form is fairly straightforward to use with designated sections that need to be completed:

Pay Payment of £19 is asked for upon completing and submitting your application.

UCAS Track This online system allows you to track your application. It will show you your final offers/rejections. Interviews will not normally appear on the system and medical schools will instead contact you with information through post or email.

UCAS Form Sections
• Personal Details (completed upon registration)
•Student Finance Details
•Course Choices
•Education
•Employment
•Personal Statement
•Reference (completed by your school)

School Reference

The role that the reference from your school plays in the application process differs between medical schools. Some include it and score it in their application process while others disregard it completely. Regardless of how it is scored it is important that you receive as positive a reference as possible to maximise your chances of receiving an offer.

The best way to get a great reference is to work hard at school and to ask a teacher that you know will only have positive things to say about you.

Together with providing the medical school with an honest report of why you are a strong applicant the reference can also help to explain any areas of weakness in your application. This might include low grades due to an illness or bereavement or explaining a disability. You only have limited space to get everything in to your personal statement so the reference is an important adjunct.

Getting the Reference You Deserve

Work Hard It goes without saying that the reference will reflect your work during the school year and if you have demonstrated hard work and determination your teacher will find it much easier to write something positive.

Ask the Right Person You will likely know some teachers better than others and some may be experienced in writing references. Make sure you ask someone you know has your best interests at heart and is able to concisely recount your best attributes.

Discuss the Reference with Them When asking for a reference, make sure you take a list of everything that you have done to get into medical school. Provide the teacher with a copy of your personal statement so that they know as much about you as possible. You can even ask for some feedback on your personal statement at the same time.

PERSONAL STATEMENT BASICS

Together with exam grades, the UCAS personal statement forms the main way that medical schools will select applicants for interview.

The personal statement gives you a limited space to explain why a medical school should invite you to interview and allows you to describe why you deserve to become a doctor.

The biggest hurdle you will need to overcome is knowing how to get started with the personal statement. We recommend attacking the personal statement in four phases:

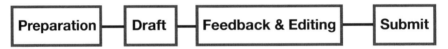

| Preparation | Draft | Feedback & Editing | Submit |

Below are some general tips to consider before getting started and then we will look at each of the above phases in detail to help you structure your personal statement.

Insider Tip

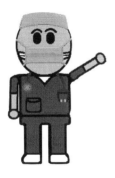

"Get started early. Not knowing where to start and wanting to write the 'perfect' personal statement first time causes you to put it off. JUST DO IT. Read past personal statements, start writing, see what happens and then edit. Even after editing two or three times coming back to your draft after a week's break will likely reveal even more edits."

Personal Statement Top Tips

Get Started Early The best way to ensure that your personal statement is as good as it possibly can be is to get started on it early. UCAS applications may be submitted from mid-September and we advise having a draft version completed at least 1 month prior to this, around the start of August.

Preparation Understanding how the personal statement is marked, knowing what to include and how to link experiences to qualities of doctor will give you a good idea of how to structure and approach the personal statement.

Divide After planning what you want to include divide the personal statement into bite-size chunks with subheadings. This will allow you to focus on different aspects such as why you want to study medicine, work experience and extracurricular activities.

Deadlines Set yourself deadlines for planning, completing each section and having a draft copy and final copy completed. This will help you stay on track and help you plan your time.

Feedback Get as many people as possible to read your personal statement. Friends and family are best for checking spelling and grammar while teachers and doctors will be best at looking at content.

Save Drafts Edit drafts multiple times to get the most concise, best final product. Make sure you save your work with whichever word processor you are using and don't lose any of your hard work.

Maximise Space UCAS set a 47 line or 4000 character limit (whichever is reached first) for you to write your personal statement.

Submit It Early Getting the personal statement in early will maximise your chances of being shortlisted for interview

Preparation

The first step in writing your personal statement is to do some research and understand what the medical schools will be looking for and how the personal statements are marked. Then you can devise a timeframe for collecting together your ideas and writing the first draft.

How Is It Marked?

Different medical schools will have different ways that they incorporate your personal statement into your overall application score. Some will give you a breakdown of their scoring criteria for entry on their admission website and others will be more vague.

Regardless of how the personal statement contributes to the overall score the scoring of the personal statement reflects how well you show a desire to study medicine, how well you demonstrate you have the skills required to be a doctor and how well you sell yourself as an individual to the medical school.

Marking will be done by local doctors and trained admission staff at the medical school. Generally speaking, the markers will want to see if the candidate has:

Do You Have What It Takes?
A realistic interest in Medicine?
Knowledge of a career in Medicine?
Demonstrated a commitment to helping others?
Demonstrated a wide range of interests?
Contributed to school/college/community activities?
A range of personal achievements (excluding exams)?

Your UCAS form and personal statement will be read and marked against a set pro-forma such as the one outlined below:

Academic Ability (/10)	Commitment to Medicine (/10)
• Predicted/actual grades • Number of subjects • Academic prizes/distinctions	• Strong reason for studying medicine • Demonstrates interest and enthusiasm • Appropriate hospital work experience • Appropriate voluntary work experience
Suitability to Medicine (/10)	Insight into Medicine (/10)
• Demonstrates reflective learning from work experience • Demonstrates understanding of the qualities of a doctor • Appreciates the highs and lows of life as a doctor	• Demonstrates interests outside of school and medicine • Relates extracurricular skills to medicine

Scoring well on the personal statement is as much about knowing what the markers are looking for as it is about your achievements and writing style. Make sure you search the admission websites for the medical schools that you are applying for to see if they outline their marking criteria. The UCAS website also offers a good insight into how the medical personal statement is marked.

As markers are looking for set criteria it is logical to structure your personal statement in a way that facilitates the scoring process. For example many students begin by stating why they want to study medicine then talk about their work experience and what they have done to pursue a career in medicine before talking about any extracurricular or personal attributes that relate to working as a doctor.

The key to scoring highly is not only stating what you have done but also reflecting on your experiences and stating how these make you suitable to be a doctor.

Statements: Being Generic Vs Being Specific

Generic

"I shadowed an F1 doctor in a busy surgical department at my local hospital for three weeks during the summer."

Specific

"Shadowing an F1 doctor on a general surgical ward taught me the importance of being organised and prioritising tasks while not being afraid to ask for help or delegate jobs when things get busy."

Generic

"I completed a Duke of Edinburgh Gold award demonstrating my leadership skills."

Specific

"I demonstrated strong leadership and teamwork skills when acting as team leader during my Duke of Edinburgh Gold expedition. I will take these skills forward when working in a multidisciplinary team and collaborating with colleagues."

Clearly stating what you have learned from specific work experience and extracurricular activities and relating this to the qualities of a doctor will score you the highest marks.

When Should I Start?

While it can be tough to motivate yourself to sit down and start planning your personal statement after exams, during the summer and before your final year of school this is probably the best time to get started.

By this time, if you followed the advice in the Work Experience Chapter of this book, you should already have some work experience and courses under your belt and plenty of things to demonstrate a desire to pursue medicine.

We recommend aiming to get a draft done by the beginning of August so you should be starting to plan your personal statement in mid-July.

Qualities of a Doctor

Doing your homework and understanding the qualities that a doctor should possess are key. Any examples you use should relate to these qualities and many are seen as 'buzz words' to use in the personal statement.

The GMC website (www.gmc.org) has further information of what attributes they expect doctors to possess.

Example Personal Statements

UCAS utilise plagiarism software to check that your personal statement is your own and has not been copied from a previous applicant or from a website. It is important that you use your own examples and wording to give you the best chance of scoring well.

Despite this you may wish to ask current medical students if you can have a look at the personal statements that they used. This will give you an objective idea of how to lay out your personal statement and help you to understand what scores well.

HOW TO WRITE THE BEST PERSONAL STATEMENT

Getting Started: Map It Out

A good way to begin is to draw a mind map on a piece of paper or using an iPad app listing the sections you wish to divide your personal statement into. We would suggest:

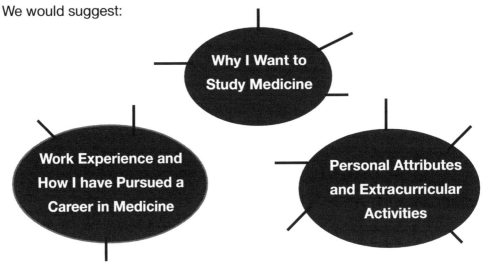

Within each of these headings you can make lists of all the things that you might like to include. This is a great way to brainstorm ideas and allows you to add extra things in at a later stage. Once you have your ideas together you can then begin to write your draft personal statement.

Draft: Just Do It

Putting your thoughts into writing can be tricky and some are better at writing than others. It is important that you get stuck in and write down anything to get started. Remember you will be editing this draft on a number of occasions before reaching the final version. Do not worry if you exceed the character or line limit set by UCAS, the draft can be edited later to get down to 47 lines or 4000 characters.

The Beginning

The first and last sentences of the personal statement are arguably the most important parts. Markers will have read thousands of personal statements many of which begin 'I want to study medicine due to a love of science and...' this can be monotonous and having an original, well-worded and passionate opening gambit can make them take notice.

The first few lines should tell the story of why you want to study medicine. This should be personal and use specific examples from your past to reflect how they influenced your career choice. This could be anything from a time that you were a patient, to visiting a relative in hospital, to work experience, to reading an exciting medical story in a book or the news.

A strong opening might draw upon some of the qualities of a doctor being reasons to go to medical school.

Example Openings

"When I was fourteen my younger brother fractured his wrist. I was captivated by how doctors and surgeons diagnosed the fracture using X-rays took him to theatre, reduced the fracture, applied a cast and discharged him within twenty-four hours. The impact their speed, communication, empathy and technical skills had on my entire family was overwhelming and I knew I wanted to have an opportunity to do the same."

"After experiencing the NHS as a patient to have a birth mark removed I understood how scientific knowledge, dexterity and empathy used by doctors can greatly improve both self-confidence and quality of life for patients."

"My natural affinity for science subjects combined with seeing the impact a hip replacement had on my grandmother's quality of life instantly made me want to become a doctor."

The Middle

The middle section of your personal statement should cover your work experience and personal attributes. Your work experience should demonstrate an understanding of the NHS and the pros and cons of being a doctor together with showing your enthusiasm and determination for going to medical school. You should show how your personal attributes and extracurricular activities will help you when studying medicine and as a doctor and this is also an opportunity for you to stand out and sell yourself with qualities such as leadership, determination, empathy, teamwork and communication skills taking a front seat.

A common pitfall for applicants is to simply list their attributes or work experience. The key to scoring highly is to reflect on your work experience, noting how certain scenarios made you feel, and stating how attributes such as leadership, that you may have developed doing something like Duke of Edinburgh, will help you as a doctor.

The End

Ending the personal statement can be tricky. You want to end on a high note and leave a good feeling about yourself with the marker. Having a summary sentence is not always necessary and it is fine to end with another example of what a fantastic doctor you will make. Below are a few tips on how to end the personal statement effectively:

Summary Statements While not necessary these do have the advantage of bringing together the driving points behind why you want to study medicine and what you are passionate about.

Link to the Beginning The last few lines can reflect the start of your personal statement and bring things together. For example in the previous student example of experiencing his grandmother's hip surgery being a driving force to study medicine a final line might be:

"(Following work experience) I now understand that elective hip surgery is only behind cataract surgery in the World Health Organisation's quality adjusted life years (QALYs) table and am passionate about studying medicine so that I might help improve the lives of others just as my grandmother's life was. "

Interests and Topical Events The ending is a good time to highlight your knowledge of medical training and topical medical stories. For example you may like to explain how you are particularly interested in.

Feedback and Editing

Once you have written your first draft to a standard that you are happy with, email the personal statement to friends, family or teachers and take a break from writing. Feedback from others might be general, might highlight some spelling or grammatical errors or, if you are lucky, give you specific tips for rewriting and improvement.

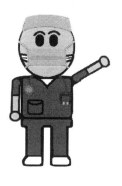

Insider Tip

"It is important that you ask people to be critical as while being told it 'looks great!' may boost your confidence it is not helpful for improving the personal statement. Don't take criticism to heart, all feedback offers learning points, and select what you believe are useful changes. Coming back to the personal statement yourself after a few days is also very helpful as you may re-read it and change points or make wording more concise."

Advice From Admission Tutors

Below are some tips from university admission tutors on how to ensure you write the best personal statement possible.

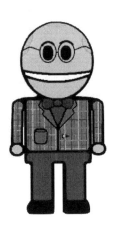

Style The overall tone of your personal statement should be positive and give the marker the impression that you are excited and interested in becoming a doctor. Your punctuation and paragraph style should remain consistent throughout.

Content The content should follow a logical structure that facilitates the scoring process (such as the one above). Unique and specific examples should be followed by reflection and thought-provoking discussion and linked to the qualities of a doctor such as empathy, communication and teamwork. It is important that you show appreciation of patients and other team members and do not just talk about doctors. When discussing the qualities of a doctor these should be backed up by specific examples form your work experience.

Show Enthusiasm and Interest The best way to demonstrate enthusiasm and a strong commitment to medicine is to use specific examples of things that interest you. This might seem obvious but a work experience placement that you enjoyed or an interest in a new type of treatment for a disease are good examples. It is important to show that you went the extra mile either by reading around the subject or organising some extra work experience.

Power Words The words you select to convey meaning are critically important in the personal statement.

For example 'I am interested in medicine' and 'I am passionate about medicine' are two very different statements conveying the same thing. During the editing process try to think about which words can be replaced to give statements more power and impact and make you sound determined and unstoppable in your active pursuit of medicine. If you are struggling a list of power words that may improve your statements is provided below.

Repetition Try not to reuse examples or repeat anything in the limited space. Every sentence should bring something new to the overall statement whether it be reflection, an example of work experience or an extracurricular activity.

Targeting Medical Schools Your personal statement will be read by each of your four medical schools. While it is not advisable to put all your eggs in one basket by stating that you like a particular type of course or university you can demonstrate an interest in research or a topical subject specific to your first choice of medical school without alienating the other three.

For example if your first choice medical school has recently opened a simulation centre, is conducting research into medical simulation or has just published an article in a medical journal on simulation this statement might read something similar to:

> " I understand the time constraints on clinical teaching in medical training and am interested in the use of simulation, I particularly enjoyed reading a recent article in the BMJ on its current applications in laparoscopic surgery. "

To the markers from the other three medical schools this is simply demonstrating a specific interest and shows enthusiasm and awareness of current training issues that you learned from your work experience.

To the marker from the medical school with the brand new simulation centre this not only shows interest but may also highlight that you have researched that medical school or at the very least makes a subconscious link to their institution.

In this way you can try to target your first choice medical school while not harming your chances with the remaining three. A good place to start is the website of your top medical school which will often list news articles about current research and developments.

Planting Questions In the same manner as targeting medical schools you may also wish to plant specific interests, such as the above interest in simulation, knowing that interviewers may well pick up on this statement and ask you about it at the interview. While not all medical school interviews will have your personal statement in front of them on the day interviewers at medical schools that do will often ask you to expand on points such as these.

Everything Counts Think carefully about everything that you write in the personal statement. If the interviewers have your personal statement in front of them anything written within it is fair game for a question. If you have made a statement about enjoying seeing a lumbar puncture being performed during neurology work experience it is only sensible to make sure you read up on the procedure and know the basics about how and why it was performed. This avoids any awkward moments when you realise that you do not fully understand something that you have included in the personal statement.

Save and Spell Check While basic it can be a nightmare if you spend a day writing your personal statement only for your computer to restart and you lose all your work. It can be equally embarrassing if you submit your final application only to later notice you have misspelled a disease name.

Chapter 2 The Interview

The medical school interview is the final and most important step in the application process. Interviews can be daunting and it is vital that you practice answering common questions and understand what the interviewers are looking for.

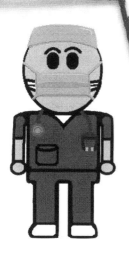

INTERVIEW OVERVIEW

The medical school interview is the final step in the medical school selection process and the face-to-face format can make it the most intimidating.

Medical schools want to select doctors of the future who have excellent communication skills, demonstrate empathy and are able to answer questions in a logical and well-reasoned fashion.

This chapter is written by a medical school admissions interviewer and covers the different formats of medical school interview used by UK medical schools, offers tips on how to best prepare for the interview and offers some examples of commonly asked questions for you to practice.

The Format

Traditionally medical school interviews consisted of a 10-20 minute interview with 2-4 interviewers asking the candidate questions. While some medical schools continue to use this tried and tested format an increasing number are utilising the Multiple Mini-Interview (MMI) format. MMI is thought to be useful as it is less time-consuming than the traditional format and universities are able to interview a larger number of applicants. The format also means that more interviewers assess the applicant helping to further standardise the process and different domains such as empathy, reasoning and personal attributes can be assessed separately at different stations.

Confusingly the number of stations and timings of interviews also differ between medical schools. It is important that you check the admissions website of the medical schools, to ensure you fully understand the format, timings and mark scheme for the interviews that you will be attending.

Traditional Interviews

The traditional interview is used in fields outside of medicine and you may have had experience of being interviewed for a part-time job or for work experience.

Medical school interviews using the traditional format last between 15-45 minutes and consist of an interview panel of 2-4 interviewers asking you a selection of questions.

The interview will begin once you walk in though the door of the interview room. The interviewers will greet you, sit opposite you on the other side of a table and begin by introducing themselves and offering a brief summary of how the interview will be conducted.

Interviewers will have a set question list, as devised by the medical school, to ask each applicant. An interviewer will typically ask you the first question, which may be very broad such as 'why medicine?', 'tell me about yourself' or 'tell me about your work experience'.

Interviewers will then probe you by asking follow on questions. As there is no buzzer or set timing for each question interviewers may wish to spend longer on some questions than others and push the best students to test their knowledge.

Some questions will be fact based such as 'what work experience have you done?', while others may test your reasoning skills with an ethical scenario.

Multiple Mini Interviews (MMI)

This is a relatively new format of interview, pioneered at McMaster University for Canadian medical school applications.

The MMI typically consists of five to ten timed stations through which you will rotate. At each station, you will be presented with a question, scenario or task. The stations usually last between 5-10 minutes and are manned by one or two interviewers.

Some MMIs include a 'rest' station to allow you to have a break at a point in the circuit.

The question, scenario or task will either be written on a laminated piece of paper or explained to you by the interviewer. The written or spoken information will usually be short, a sentence or two, outlining the question, scenario or task and what is required from you. Stations testing empathy, communication skills and integrity may feature an actor with whom you will be interacting for the task or scenario.

How You Will Be Assessed At MMI

★ Reasons for application to study medicine

★ Influence of work experience

★ Contribution to school and society

★ Academic ability and intellect

★ Knowledge of the course and medical careers

★ Descriptive skills

★ Dexterity

★ Empathy

★ Communication skills

★ Initiative and coping under pressure

★ Reasoning and problem solving skills

★ Leadership and team work skills

On a practical level the process will start with a bell or buzzer sounding to indicate you may start your first station. You may then read or listen to the interviewer give you the question, scenario or task. You will then have the remaining time (usually 5-10 minutes) in which to give your answer. A second bell or buzzer will sound to indicate when your time at that station is up. You will then have 1-2 minutes of time in which to move to your next station before another buzzer sounds indicating you can start your next station on the circuit.

Each interviewer will give you a mark for their station with transferrable skills such as communication, confidence and judgment under pressure scored at each station and aggregated.

Oxbridge Interviews

The interviews utilised by Oxford and Cambridge are a little different to those employed by other universities. You may have heard rumours or examples of applicants being asked increasingly bizarre questions or handed something like a brick and being asked what they would do with it. For the most part these are simply rumours from days gone by however the format of the Oxbridge interview is much less scripted than other medical schools. Interviewers will still be interested in why you want to study medicine at Oxbridge and what work experience you have done but there will be no set questions to ask rather interviewers will allow a conversation to naturally develop within the time frame.

Oxbridge interviews will focus on problem solving and theoretical discussion and are more likely to pick questions that stem from information included in your personal statement. Interviewers are more interested in how you go about solving or discussing a problem or question than you getting the right answer to the point that they may not even know the correct answer themselves!

Generally speaking you will still be asked the common questions as outlined later on in this chapter but you should expect more discussion and a need to think outside the box than at other medical school interviews.

Assessment Centres

A few medical schools such as Warwick employ what they term an 'assessment centre' or 'assessment day'. This essentially involves a short traditional interview, tour of the school and may also involve a group task.

Group tasks involve you discussing a topic with your peers while assessors score you based on team work and communication.

FAQs

Who is on the Interview Panel?

Whichever format of interview you attend the interviewers will be current medical school staff and doctors form local hospitals. All interviewers should have undergone training on how to conduct the interview and fairly score candidates.

In practical terms it will not matter if the person interviewing you is a surgeon, an anaesthetist, the medical school dean or a neonatologist. They will have set questions to ask and the only difference it will make is that will be less likely to fall asleep if you show interest in work experience undertaken in their field.

How is the Interview Scored?

The exact scoring system used differs between each medical school.

In general, each question will be scored by the interviewers on a scale, such as 1-10. Characteristics such as confidence, maturity and communication skills will be assessed throughout the interview and scored independently.

At the end of the interview scores will be added up and compared to other students in that interview group. Some medical schools have a set score for offering a place while others ask for the top three to four applicants in a group to be offered places others combine interview and UCAS scores before ranking applicants and making offers.

When Will I Get The Results?

Typically medical schools will submit their scores to UCAS within two weeks of the interview and UCAS will then process these and notify students. Due to the volume of applicants do not worry if you don't hear back immediately and some medical school offers may be issued long after the interview itself. If you are worried check both the university admissions website, interview documentation and UCAS website to see what the policy for announcing offers is at the schools that you have applied to.

PREPARING FOR INTERVIEW

You may have been interviewed for a part-time job but for many students university interviews will be the first experience of the interview process. This will be the first of many interviews in your career and once you appreciate that preparation is key much of the anxiety surrounding the process will disappear.

Preparation for most interviews can be divided into long-term and short-term preparation. Long term is everything you do to bolster your personal statement while short term is focussed on interview practise and technique.

Do Your Research

As previously mentioned the precise interview format, timing and scoring will vary between each medical school. It is important that you check the website of each medical school well in advance so that you are prepared for how you will be interviewed.

Most medical schools have descriptions of their interview process on their admissions websites and some go as far as to tell you how you will be scored.

Interviews typically range from 15 minutes to 1 hour depending on the format. Finding out how long the interview will be is helpful to give you an idea of how succinct your answers need to be. For example some MMI stations are only five minutes in length with strict timings as you will have to move on to the next station.

Another way to find out about the interview process is to ask school leavers or friends who may have had interviews at the medical school the previous year. It is also useful to ask current medical students and doctors at open days and during your work experience to provide you with further insight into the process.

It is also advisable to research how you will get to and from the interview venue and whether you will travel to the university the night before and stay in the city to avoid delays. This may involve booking train tickets and accommodation and finding out where exactly the interview will be held.

Practise Questions

Practice makes perfect and it is important that you practise your interview technique and how you will address the common questions. While there is no way to prepare for every question that might be asked it is sensible to prepare the most common questions and have a framework with which to answer the more difficult questions.

Long Term Preparation	Short Term Preparation
★ A-Levels ★ Work experience ★ Volunteering ★ Attending courses ★ Collecting medical news stories ★ Writing a solid personal statement	★ Researching the interview format ★ Preparing how you will answer questions ★ Practising your interview technique ★ Writing out personalised answers

In the subsequent chapters you will find some of the commonly recurring questions that are asked repeatedly at medical school interviews. Frameworks are used for you to add your own experiences. Nearer the time try to set up formal interview practise with someone outside the family (and preferably with a medical background). Put on your smart 'interview' attire and treat the mock interview like the real thing. This provides realistic interview practise and tests how you perform under pressure. It should also make the real thing seem slightly less scary.

INTERVIEW TECHNIQUE

Being 'good' at interviews is a skill and as with all skills it will get better with understanding how to improve and then practising. Studies have shown that impressing interviewers and scoring highly at interviews is as much about how you communicate and convey you answer as much as it is about the content of the answer itself.

Communication Skills

Interviews are not just about facts and it is important that you are aware of other factors that will contribute to your interview score and the overall impression that you leave the interviewers with.

Body Language

Body language is extremely important and plays a pivotal role in effective communication. It can be difficult to know how to sit, who to look at or what to do with your arms during an interview.

Sitting A number of studies have identified the position of sitting slightly forward feet planted on the ground with hands crossed or fingers locked and forearms resting on your thighs as being the optimum position for interviews. This position makes you look calm and ready and is in between leaning over the table and slouching back in your chair. This position can be maintained for the majority of the interview and allows you to sit back slightly between questions or at the end of the interview.

Smile Smiling has been shown to increase attractiveness by a factor of ten and will also convey confidence and personality to the interviewers. While you may be extremely nervous make sure you smile when you greet the panel and try to show enthusiasm when talking about why you want to study medicine or something that you are passionate about.

Eye Contact Ensure that you make eye contact with the interviewers from the start. If you find holding eye contact difficult practice focussing on peoples' eyebrows when you talk to them (the eye of the other person cannot discriminate whether you are looking at their eye or eyebrow due to proximity). When listening to questions concentrate on the interviewer asking the questions nodding to show understanding. When giving your answers make sure you make eye contact with all the panel and not just the interviewer asking the question. At least one of the interviewers will be making notes or scoring you so don not be phased if they do not maintain eye contact.

Hands From the initial handshake to using hand gestures to enforce points your hands help to demonstrate confidence and conviction if used correctly. Upon entering the room respond to handshakes if offered and look the interviewers in the eyes. Keep you hands on your knees or lap when listening to questions and raise them when making a firm point.

Appearance For male applicants: smart shoes, smart suit, plain shirt and plain tie. For women a smart skirt or trousers and a shirt with or without a suit jacket will be fine. It is important that you appear smart and dress as a doctor would when seeing patients in a clinic.

Active Listening When being asked questions sit attentively. Movements such as tilting your head or nodding in understanding demonstrate active listening and will make you appear more engaging to the interviewers.

Communicating Effectively

Once you have mastered body language it is time analyse how you deliver your responses to the interviewers as an excellent answer delivered in a quiet, stuttering manner will score less well than one given with gusto.

Clarity Project your voice beyond the interviewers, sit upright and speak clearly. You will be nervous initially and may hear your voice waiver. This is entirely normal and you will settle in to things after you begin speaking.

Length of Response Stopping yourself from talking when nervous can be extremely difficult however interviewers are likely to lose concentration after around 3 minutes of hearing you talk. Most structured points can be given within 2-3 minutes leaving time for further questions.

Speed Some people talk quickly others talk slowly. Try to find a balance and don't be afraid to pause to consider the question before jumping into your answer.

Vocal Tonality The sentence 'I want to be a doctor' can be interpreted in a number of ways depending on the tonality of the delivery. For instance a person increasing their inflection towards the end of the sentence suggests a question: 'I want to be a doctor?'. While delivery with a firm tone suggests more of a statement: 'I want to be a doctor!'. More over emphasis of words can dramatically alter the sentence structure; 'I WANT to be a doctor', 'I want to BE A DOCTOR'. Changing your inflection and emphasising words prevents interviewers from getting bored. Think about how quickly you lose interest when speaking to someone talking about something in a monotonous, single tone voice and then think about someone who changes their tone and emphasises words. Less easy to fall asleep, right?.

Enthusiasm Following on from tonality and word emphasis make sure that you are enthusiastic when delivering your answers. Smiling and tonality make up a large portion of this the rest is about overcoming nerves and remembering that you should be excited about becoming a doctor and the things that you have done.

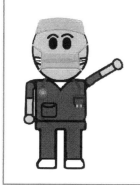

Insider Tip

"Try altering your vocal tonality and word emphasis and practise improving your eye-contact by looking at eyebrows. You can do this right now!."

Interview Frameworks

Although you cannot predict and prepare for every question that might be asked at interview it is helpful to have a framework to answer specific types of questions. Roughly speaking questions asked at any type of interview can be categorised into motivational, situational, judgement and ethical.

Having a framework will help you to logically structure your answers for both basic and more challenging questions and help you think under pressure. Different question types will require different frameworks. Question types fall into categories or domains based on what the interviewers are testing. Whichever framework you use you should be able to cut your answer down to 3-4 solid, personal experiences and reflect on each.

Motivational and Experiential: CAPS

e.g. Why Medicine? Why This Medical School? Tell me About Your Work Experience

Clinical

Academic

Personal

Skills

Problem Solving: SEAS

e.g. One of your friends is consistently late for lectures and struggles with work. What would you do?

Seek Information

Empathy

Action

Seek Help

Skills Questions: STAR

e.g. How have you shown leadership? Have you been part of a team?

Situation

Task

Action

Result

You can find examples of these frameworks in action in the next three chapters.

MMI Technique

MMIs are significantly different from the traditional interview, becoming familiar with the structure, logic and expectations of a MMI will better prepare you for your interview.

The Circuit It is important to remember that you will be rotating around a circuit with other students behind and ahead of you and it can be easy to be distracted by loud interviewers or applicants, especially if the MMI is conducted in a large hall.

Read The Question Ensure you read or listen to each question and understand what the interviewers want from your answer

Time Management Make sure your answers are succinct and focussed. Time is limited as you will be moving stations and there will be little time to waffle on.

Don't Panic If a station goes badly forget about it and give the next station your best shot

Actors Try to treat the actors seriously and listen and respond to their scenarios. You will be assessed on your empathy and communication skills so ensure you employ the active listening suggestions listed above in the communication skills section and use phrases such as 'I understand', 'I am sure that must be difficult for you', 'I am sorry to hear that' to directly demonstrate empathy and understanding.

Content

Regardless of the interview type, medical schools will want to know about your work experience, your extracurricular activities, how you deal with pressure, how you resolve problems and whether you can demonstrate empathy.

Be Personal and Specific Talking about generic things like 'I saw a patient having blood taken' or 'I have leadership skills' will not score you as many points as using personal experiences and reflecting on what you learned.

Structure Your Answers Structuring your answers into 3-4 headlines will make it easy for interviewers to follow and prevent you from wasting time with waffle.

Common Questions Write out example answers for common questions and then practise them. Try not to be too scripted rather work on your delivery and enthusiasm once you are happy with your content.

Use Your Personal Statement Interviewers may not have access to or may not have read your personal statement. Make sure that you talk about all the best points that you have written down and do not assume that the interviewers have read it. Your personal statement should be structured to say why you want to do medicine, what work experience you have done and what you do outside of work; these are also three of the most commonly asked questions!

Show Your Working For tough ethical or decision-making questions be sure to talk through what you are thinking. There is often no right or wrong answer rather the interviewers want to see you logically discussing both sides of the argument or problem.

Be Positive and Sell, Sell, Sell Interviewers want to hear how great you are and it is important that you are not bashful or reserved when telling them about your achievements and why they should choose you. Turn everything into a positive and don't undersell yourself.

Don't Give An Overview Outlining how you are going to answer a question or explaining your framework is unnecessary and risky. One particularly awkward moment occurred when an interview candidate confidently stated there were three reasons he wanted to be a medic only for him to be unable to recall the third!

Read The Instructions MMI stations will often provide you with written information either before or upon approaching the station. Traditional interviews may also provide you with a written scenario to discuss. Whatever the situation remain calm and read the instructions or scenario carefully. Try to mentally highlight the important points and understand what they want you to do.

Answer The Question This might seem silly but it is amazing how often candidates do not give a direct answer or go off-topic. Make sure you understand what has been asked and avoid giving a long-winded introduction.

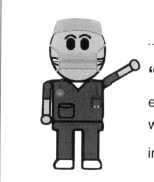

Insider Tip

"Use specific, personal examples from your work experience to help answer challenging questions. This will keep the interviewers engaged and demonstrate insight into medicine."

Other Factors

The thought of the interview can be scary and there are some other variables that you will need to consider such as how you are going to get to the venue and what happens when you get there. Most medical schools will send you detailed information regarding the interview process and venue in good time. Below are some top tips for how to stay calm around the time of the interview.

The Night Before You may have chosen to stay in the city before your interview or you may be travelling up on the day. Whatever you have chosen to do ensure that you have your clothes prepared, shoes shined and know where and when you need to be at the interview location. If the medical school has asked you to bring anything with you to the interview, such as identification, make sure that you have it ready to take. Relax and get a good night's sleep, making sure you set your alarm to wake up in good time the next morning.

On the Day Get up in good time and have a proper breakfast. Make sure you factor in traffic if you are driving to the interview location. Most students will travel with their parents and it is up to you whether you allow them to come with you to the interview registration or force them to stay in the car or a café!

Upon arriving at the venue you will need to register so that the organisers know that you have arrived. Occasionally your interview time slot may have been altered. If this is the case don't panic and go with the flow. There will be refreshments provided and you will be told where you can wait before the interview.

An interviewer or facilitator will usually call you in once they are ready. Upon entering greet and shake hands with the interviewers ensuring that you try to appear as confident as possible. The interviewers will then show you to your seat, ready to begin.

What The Interviewers Say

We asked a selection of medical school interviewers to give their opinions on what makes the difference between a good candidate and an excellent candidate. Here is what they had to say.

"The biggest challenge of any interview candidate is

answering the questions posed in a way that incorporates your best points in a concise format. In traditional and, in particular, in MMI interviews your time to tell the interviewers how fantastic you are is limited. This can be especially difficult when asked a very broad, open

question such as 'Why should we choose you?'."

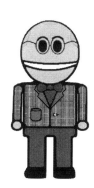

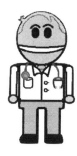

"As a medical school interviewer I can tell you that the best

candidates are the ones who answer the questions posed in a logical and structured format and who have clearly thought

about how they will answer the common questions."

"Candidates who appear confident, with good body

language and vocal intonation have often acquired this through previous interview or public speaking experiences. The more formal interview practice that you do the more relaxed you will be on the day of the real thing and this will

translate into a more confident performance."

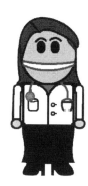

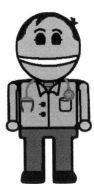

"Ask any interviewer what separates the best and worst interview candidates and they are likely to respond with a single word 'waffle'. (Most) interviewers are human and will be interviewing students for the entire day of interviews. Think about the last time you spoke with someone, maybe a friend or relative, who told a long and boring story. It can be difficult to stay focused and retain information when candidates talk for longer than 3-4 minutes or repeat themselves. Preparing and practising questions with a set framework will help you to get across your best selling points in a concise format."

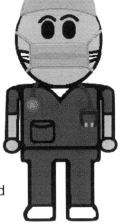

"Some candidates struggle to sell themselves and feel awkward or boastful when asked why they would be a good doctor or why they should be chosen. The best way around this is to bring objectivity into the answer.

For example: Rather than saying 'I am a great leader' you may be more comfortable saying 'feedback from my teachers and peers highlights my strong leadership skills'. You should of course back this up with a specific example such as when you captained a sports team or led a Duke of Edinburgh expedition."

Chapter 3 Traditional Interview Questions

Most traditional medical school interviews last 10-30 minutes and interviewers will take turns asking motivational and scenario-based questions

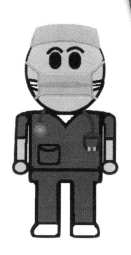

WHY DO YOU WISH TO STUDY MEDICINE?

This is a fairly easy and predictable question and is often the first question asked by interviewers. Despite this it is a broad, open question and candidates may waffle.

The answer to this question is likely to be the first paragraph of your personal statement. Remember to assume that the interviewers have not read your personal statement and don't be afraid to structure your answer in a similar manner.

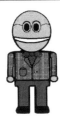

Interviewers Are Looking For:
Commitment to Medicine; ability to communicate; self-confidence and enthusiasm; motivation and determination to study and realistic reasons for choice.

Your answer should be structured into three or four key points and use specific examples. This question lends itself to the **CAPS** framework. Below you will find some ideas to help get you started creating a personalised response.

Clinical Reasons

Have you or a family member been a hospital patient? Do you now want to give something back? A clinical story can often be a good way to start and helps to gain the interviewers' attention and get them to invest in you. Other clinical reasons might include:

★ The variety of illnesses and patients
★ The ability to immediately diagnose and help someone
★ The huge affect certain treatments can make to a patient's quality of life e.g. cataract surgery or hip and knee replacements.
★ Mix of acute and chronic illnesses
★ Mix of ward, clinic, operating work

Academic Reasons

Academic doesn't just mean top A-Levels, a career in medicine will stimulate you intellectually and offer opportunities to learn and teach others.

★ Challenging

★ Enjoy lifelong learning

★ Problem-solving when assessing patients

★ Knowledge can be applied to help others

★ Research and potential to advance areas of medicine

★ Opportunities to teach others

Personal Reasons

This can be linked to your clinical reasons if you have a personal story of experiencing healthcare.

★ Enjoy working under pressure

★ Enjoy responsibility

★ Enjoy teamwork

★ Enjoy talking with patients and helping others

★ Job satisfaction

Skills Reasons

Doctors must have strong communication, organisation, teamwork, leadership and management skills

★ No other job combines practical skills with knowledge and interpretation

★ Enjoy learning/good at practical skills

★ Learning surgical procedures is fun and surgery can instantly help patients

Example Answers

> **"**I enjoy science subjects at school and want to help others using these skills. Doctors are well respected and I like talking with patients and learning new things. I think there is no better career than medicine and I can see myself working as a doctor...**"**

Analysis: Poor Answer.

The candidate has started with a very generic statement, used weak wording and hasn't used any specific examples.

> **"** When I was 14 my brother fractured his wrist playing football. The orthopaedic surgeons reduced the fracture in theatre and applied a cast before discharging my brother within 24hours. Seeing the use of technology, communication skills and operative skills vastly improve my brother's life made me want to pursue a career in medicine and fitted in nicely with my strong academic record in science subjects at school...**"**

Analysis: Strong Answer.

This example is a good opening using specific examples to highlight insight into medicine and a drive to become a doctor. The story element grips the interviewer from the start and shows that you understand a patient's journey. It can be expanded on by looking in detail at the qualities of a doctor and the question of 'why a doctor rather than a nurse?' can be incorporated into it.

WHY BECOME A DOCTOR RATHER THAN A NURSE OR PHYSIOTHERAPIST?

Following on from the above question it is important that you make a distinction between healthcare professionals and the role and qualities of a doctor. Try not to say anything too negative about other healthcare professionals but be sure to draw a wide distinction between their roles and the roles of a doctor.

A good way to answer this question is to begin by outlining the key differences and then use a specific example from your work experience such as a nurse or physio asking a doctor for advice on further management of a patient.

Role of a Doctor Vs Other Healthcare Professionals

- Ultimate responsibility lies with the doctor
- Doctors make clinical decision based upon medical training
- Consultants are seen as team leaders
- Postgraduate training for doctors allows wide areas of specialisation and acquisition of knowledge
- Can become a surgeon, anaesthetist, GP etc and use acquired skills to greatly impact patient care
- Doctors can affect teaching and research on a much larger scale

- Nurses and physios often specialise in certain areas, run clinics and can prescribe or assess patients with extra training. The ultimate differences are leadership, responsibility, knowledge and practical skills. While specialist nurses can have similar roles to F1 doctors they cannot progress beyond this level and they have a limited role in decision-making regarding patient care.

TELL US ABOUT YOUR WORK EXPERIENCE

You may have mentioned some of your work experiences as examples in answering why you want to study medicine. This is a further opportunity to detail what you did, how much you did, what you learned and how the experiences affected you.

If you followed the advice in our Becoming A Doctor book and kept a reflective diary or bullet points of specific experiences while on work experience now is the time to use them.

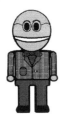

Interviewers Are Looking For:
Commitment to Medicine; informed about course and career; ability to communicate; self-confidence; enthusiasm, insight, initiative, resilience and empathy.

You will be scored not only on the type, breadth and time spent doing both voluntary and clinical work experience but also on how you reflect on this at interview.

Example Answer

"I spent 6 months volunteering at a care home for the elderly. I went there every Tuesday and Thursday evenings and spent time talking with the residents and making tea. I noticed that many of the residents were lonely and just spending time listening to their stories and sitting with them made a huge difference. The experience made me really appreciate some of the problems faced by the elderly. As the majority of hospital admissions are those at the extremes of age this experience will be invaluable when communicating with patients on elderly care wards and their families."

The **CAPS** structure can again be used to structure your own answer or you may prefer to simply use clinical work experience and voluntary work experience as headings. The key is reflecting on specific experiences and explaining.

Hospital Work Experience	Voluntary Work Experience
Clinical What department? How long? What did you see? What did you do? **Academic** What did you learn? **Personal** How did the experience affect you? **Skills** Did you learn any skills such as history taking, examination, first aid or lifesaver skills?	**Clinical** Where? How long? What was your role? **Academic** What did you learn? **Personal** How did the experience affect you? **Skills** Did you learn any skills such as history taking, examination, first aid or lifesaver skills?

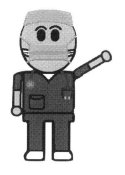

Insider Tip

"Use specific, personal examples from your work experience to help answer challenging questions. This will keep the interviewers engaged and demonstrate insight into medicine."

TELL US ABOUT AN EXTRACURRICULAR INTEREST

This is an opportunity to sell yourself as an individual, link qualities to those of a doctor and demonstrate your organisational skills.

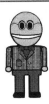

Interviewers Are Looking For:
Ability to prioritise; communication skills; enthusiasm; resilience; self-confidence; capacity to cope with a range of activities.

As the question asks for a specific example or examples you can either use the **STAR** framework or use a how, where, what, when, why method to structure your answer. Try to choose examples that will impress the interviewers and explain how you prioritised and managed you time.Any extracurricular activities area acceptable but remember to try and link them back to the qualities of a doctor and say why they will be useful when starting medicine.

Situation

• Sports Team	• Creative Writing
• Individual Sport	• DIY
• Equestrian	• Learning a language
• Musical Instrument	• Becoming a ski instructor
• Dancing	• Duke of Edinburgh Award

Task

This might include competing for a prize, attaining a grade in a musical instrument, gaining a flying license or being chosen for a regional or national team.

- What was the ultimate goal?
- What was your role in the team?

Action
- How did you practice?
- How did you fit this around schoolwork?
- Where there any setbacks?

Result
- What did you achieve?
- What did you learn from the experience?
- How will this relate to being a doctor?
- Will you be able to balance work and life at medical school and as a doctor?

Example Answer

"This year I completed my first marathon in New York running 26.2 miles in a time of 4 hours 8 minutes and raising over £1000 for the prostate cancer charity. Finishing the challenging course on behalf of a charity gave me a great sense of achievement and demonstrated that all the hard work that I had put into training over the previous six months had come to fruition. In order to prepare for the event I followed a training regime diligently and had to achieve set distances each week balanced between school work.

Running and charity work demonstrate that I hold a suitable balance between my work and personal life and that I maintain a high level of physical and mental fitness which is vital in providing patients with the best care possible."

TELL US ABOUT A CURRENT MEDICAL TOPIC THAT HAS INTERESTED YOU?

This question is based almost entirely on preparation. Bookmark interesting news articles, websites and links to journal articles. Keep a folder of cut outs from physical newspapers.

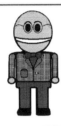

Interviewers Are Looking For:
Awareness of current developments; ability to communicate; insight, integrity and enthusiasm.

There are always plenty of news articles and research articles and it is important to choose one that genuinely interests you.

Interviewers want to know that not only are you interested in medicine but that you have gone the extra mile and read around the article, looking up any terms or points that you are unsure about. Usually a quick Wikipedia search of a medical term, disease or treatment will suffice to ensure you understand what you have read. Below are some sources to help you get started:

Student BMJ and BMJ online Registration for the student BMJ is free for some online articles or you could ask a local library or medical friend to get you the most recent issues.

New Scientist More science-based than medical but may offer some interesting articles.

Health Websites Most newspapers and news sites have dedicated health sections with editorials and articles on the latest health stories.

BMA and Royal College Websites These have news areas with links to news stories that affect members. They also offer good advice for prospective medics.

Situation

- Where and when did you read the article?
- Why did it interest you?

Task

- What did the article say?
- Who conducted the research?

Action

- What was the conclusion?
- How did it affect you?
- How did it affect medicine?

Result

- Did you look further into the article?
- Did you learn about the specific disease/treatment/microbe etc?

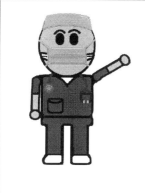

Insider Tip

"If you want to apply to a specific medical school look at the medical school research section online which will likely give links to the latest research and news articles coming out of the medical school research departments"

WHAT DO YOU KNOW ABOUT THE UNDERGRADUATE MEDICAL COURSE HERE?

Interviewers will look for evidence that the candidate has done some research about the course. Evidence for this might include the fact that the candidate recognises that the course is traditional, integrated or PBL and how the course is organised.

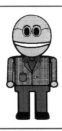

Interviewers Are Looking For:
Knowledge of the course, insight, motivation and enthusiasm

This information is easily accessible through each medical schools' website (usually under course details) or can be found in our Medical Schools Guide book. Focus on points that the medical school themselves highlight as why their course stands out from others.

The **CAPS** framework can help you to structure you answer.

Clinical
- What is the type of course
- When patient contact first happens
- Which hospitals (academies) students are sent to for clinical attachments
- When is the elective period?

Academic
- Does the school have strong research links
- When Student Selected Components (SSCs) occur
- Is there a tutor or parenting scheme for freshers?
- Is a BSc compulsory? What intercalated options are there?

Personal

- Personal motivating factors for coming to the medical school
- What is the City like?
- How big is each year?
- Are there strong university sports teams?

Skills

- Type of anatomy teaching (cadaveric/pro-sections/computer-based)
- Is there a new skills or simulated centre
- Can you study abroad on ERASMUS or combine a second language

WHAT HAPPENS AFTER YOU GRADUATE?

This question is again about preparation. The medical career path for the common specialties is widely available online and in our Becoming a Doctor book.

The easiest way to answer this question is simply to use a chronological method taking the interviewer from Foundation year one up to consultant.

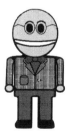

Interviewers Are Looking For:
The interviewer will look for evidence that you have some insight into issues such as the Foundation Years; GMC registration, choosing a specialty; length of training; postgraduate specialty examinations; postgraduate research and career structures.

Example Answers

> **"**After graduation doctors undertake the two-year foundation programme. At the end of F1 doctors gain full registration with the GMC. During the F2 year doctors can apply to specialist training. The length of specialist training differs between each specialty with GP taking 3 years and surgery taking around 10 years to become a consultant.**"**

Analysis: Strong answer.

This is a good start and you may then wish to focus on a career path that interests you highlighting exams and courses that may be required.

ASIDE FROM WORK EXPERIENCE AND VOLUNTARY WORK WHAT HAVE YOU DONE TO FIND OUT MORE ABOUT BEING A DOCTOR?

Most students will have been on work experience and voluntary placements prior to interview. This question gives you an opportunity to stand out and mention extra courses, placements or reading that you may have done.

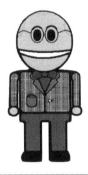

Interviewers Are Looking For:
Commitment to medicine, lateral thinking, problem solving.

Interviewers want to know that you didn't just do the bare minimum work experience to get by but are actually interested in medicine.

Commitment To Medicine
★ Reading books about the history of medicine
★ Reading medical journals such as student BMJ or BMJ
★ Attending medical lectures
★ Visiting medical/surgical museums
★ Attending practical workshops or courses
★ Talking with medical students or doctors
★ Reading medical news articles
★ Working for a charity

Remember to reflect on your examples given and to be specific.

WHAT WOULD YOU DO IF YOU DO NOT GET A PLACE THIS YEAR?

This question may catch you off-guard as it has negative undertones. The question is not suggesting you are performing poorly at interview but rather tests your motivation and determination together with demonstrating a realistic back up plan should you be unsuccessful.

Begin by demonstrating insight into the competitive nature of medicine and the importance of having a back up plan.

Make sure you state that you are determined to become a doctor and would want to gain feedback as to how your application could be improved for application the following year.

Doing further work experience, paid hospital work and volunteering will help to gain further insight into medicine and improve your chances the following year. Give specific examples and make sure you state why you think they will make you a better candidate.

WHAT IS YOUR BIGGEST WEAKNESS?

Talking about weaknesses is tricky.

The key to this question is turning your weakness into a positive and leaving the interviewers with a feeling that you have identified an area lacking in your CV or personal life and have then done something about it.

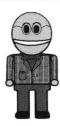

Interviewers Are Looking For:
Insight into areas for improvement, ability to be put under pressure.

Choose something that is not too much of a flaw and can be easily improved. Choosing a skill to improve moves the questions away from being too personal and allows you to give a positive spin and move to a positive note.

Example Answers

"I have high standards and like efficiency I therefore get frustrated when ... I deal with this frustration by taking a step back and remaining calm...**"**

"It is important to be aware of your weaknesses and while I feel I have a strong academic background I have not lived by myself before and this will be a challenge I look forward to when moving to university.**"**

HOW WOULD YOU DESCRIBE YOUR COMMUNICATION SKILLS?

Communication skills can be difficult to quantify, luckily feedback from teachers and talks given provide plenty of ammunition to highlight your communication skills. You can use the **STAR** framework to structure your answer.

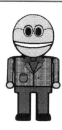

Interviewers Are Looking For:
Effective communication skills are vital for doctors and interviewers want specific examples of how your communication skills

Rather than sounding arrogant and simply talking about your communication skills try to give examples of feedback from presentation so that you provide interviewers with objective evidence.

Example Answers

> "I believe that I have excellent communication skills as demonstrated by my feedback when talking with patients as part of my hospital/voluntary work experience and when I have given presentations in school."

> "I demonstrated effective communications skills when leading my school debating society to victory in the national debating championships. This required both problem solving and listening which will be vital when explaining treatments to patients."

GIVE AN EXAMPLE OF WHEN YOU SHOWED EMPATHY TO A PATIENT?

When asked for specific examples the **STAR** framework of situation, task, action, result can help to structure your answer.

This is essentially a communication skills question and should focus on a personal example of a patient you saw on work experience or during voluntary work.

Make sure you mention how the interaction made you feel and

Example Answer

"During my regular voluntary work in a community hospital I spent time talking with an 88 year old lady who had fallen and sustained an olecranon fracture that had been treated with a plate, screws and plaster.

She was previously living independently and had not other injuries. She was unable to go directly home as the injury to her dominant hand meant that she could not manage by herself.

She was very frustrated at her lack of independence and felt that she was a burden on her family who visited her regularly.

My grandmother had been in a similar situation when she broke her hip and I sympathised with her situation and was able to explain that her family would not consider her a burden.

She was happy to have someone to talk to and I feel the experience will help me empathise with similar patients when working as a doctor "

GIVE AN EXAMPLE OF YOUR TEAMWORK SKILLS

The **STAR** framework should be employed to structure your answer. Link your example to the qualities of a good team player and reflect on the experience.

Qualities Of A Good Team Player
• **Understands their role and how it fits in with the overall team**: reliable, consistent, works hard, seeks help appropriately, takes initiative
• **Treats others with respect:** appreciates the role of others, approachable, responds to requests, allows others to perform their role, offer support when required
• **Flexible and able to compromise**: can adapt to changes, can consider different viewpoints, can compromise with other team members
• **Communicates and listens**: expresses thoughts clearly, proposes solutions not problems to the team, understands and listens to other views, accepts and acts on criticisms and feedback

Situation: Captaining school rugby team

Task: I was responsible for team mates and was required to motivate my peers when playing matches under pressure

Action: I was supportive and flexible if team mates were struggling. I listened to the coach and acted upon suggestions and improvements that they felt would help the team.

Result: This experience impressed upon me the importance of maintaining good rapport with people and our team was undefeated for the season."

GIVE AN EXAMPLE ABOUT WHEN YOU WERE A BAD TEAM MEMBER

The key to this question is stating how it changed your practice and what you learned from the experience. Do not choose an example that is too bad but rather one with a good learning point. The **STAR** framework can be used to structure the answer.

As with any 'negative' interview question ensure that you only dwell for a moment on the negativity before moving on and talking about the positive aspects of what you learned and how you improved.

Example Answer

"Prior to playing an important rugby match I had been been unwell and was not feeling 100% for the match. Despite this I was determined to play and did not tell my team mates or coach. My performance was poor and I did not contribute to the team as well as normal and missed several important conversions and was later substituted.

This taught me the importance of holding the team above my own personal desire to play. I apologised to my team mates and coach and in the future I always report any illness or injury to the coach who can make the best decision for the team when selecting players.

I will take this forward in medicine by knowing when to ask for help and understanding my own limitations to ensure patient safety"

HOW CAN DOCTORS' COMMUNICATION SKILLS INFLUENCE PATIENT CARE

This is a communication skills question and should focus on a personal example of a patient you saw on work experience. When asked for specific examples the **STAR** framework of situation, task, action, result can help to structure your answer.

Example Answer

"During my orthopaedic work experience I observed a doctor talking with a 48 year old lady with back pain.

She had a small L4/5 disc bulge but no other abnormality on MRI and was refusing to take pain relief or mobilise.

The doctor succinctly conveyed the diagnosis and treatment plan in an understandable way and encouraged the patient to mobilise with pain relief to facilitate her recovery. He also explained that she would be followed up by the musculoskeletal physios and could return if she developed any neurology.

I know this was effective as the nursing staff noted that the family were happy with the outcome and the patient began to mobilise and was discharged the following week."

HOW HAVE YOU SHOWN INTEGRITY?

This question could also be phrased 'tell us about a mistake you have made'. Integrity is the principle of being honest and is of vital importance for doctors to possess this trait. The **STAR** framework can be used to structure the answer.

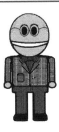

Interviewers Are Looking For:

An example of a mistake or error where the candidate subsequently takes responsibility and acts in a manner befitting of a doctor

The key to this question is stating how the mistake changed your practice and what you learned from the experience. Do not choose an example that is too bad but rather one with a good learning point.

Example Answer

"At school I was part of the young enterprises group pitching business ideas for a competition.

I was also busy doing coursework and had neglected my job as project manager and was under prepared for a group pitch after school. I made some basic errors when describing our business idea and we did not win the competition. I apologised to my tutor and took responsibility for my actions. In future I ensured that I managed my time better and sought help with task when taking on too much. I will take this forward as a doctor when mistakes can be made and it is important that these are reported and discussed openly and with honesty."

WHAT MAKES A GOOD TEACHER?

This open question may seem difficult to answer at first glance.

The key to this question is to think of the best teacher you have had and use this personal example to elaborate on the qualities they possessed.

Make sure you finish the question by emphasising that you possess these qualities and back the claim up with evidence. This is also a good time to talk about any teaching you have done yourself to younger students or as part of work experience.

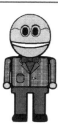

Interviewers Are Looking For:
An affinity for teaching is important as doctors at all stages of their training teach junior colleagues, patients and lay people to continue professional development and patient care.

Example Answer"

"I believe that the best teachers possess a number of characteristics such as setting goals, creating a teaching plan, defining learning styles or respecting students however from my personal experiences the three most important characteristics are enthusiasm, being a role model and reflecting on feedback. I have demonstrated these when..."

HOW DO YOU MANAGE YOUR TIME EFFECTIVELY?

Doctors are busy and it is important that you are able to demonstrate the ability to prioritise and structure your working life. This question also gives you an opportunity to talk about all the things you do outside of school and how you balance these with your school work.

Time Management Skills
Ways of managing your time might include: • Planning your work • Keeping a list/diary • Prioritising the most important tasks • Anticipating clashes and problems • Not taking on too much and knowing your limitations The main skills involved in effective time management are planning, prioritising, multitasking, working in a team, delegating work and reflecting on the result.

Begin by talking about your extracurricular activities (see previous example) and use these as examples as to how you manage your time

Organisation or management skills are similar to time management skills.

If you have organised an event or project use this as a specific example and say what you did. If you haven't organised anything describe how you organise your extracurricular activities.

How WOULD YOUR FRIENDS DESCRIBE YOU?

This question may seem difficult to answer well. The key is to demonstrate that your have made friends from from all activities that you do. For example school friends, sports team friends etc. Try to select 2-3 characteristics that are linked to the qualities of a doctor.

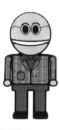

Interviewers Are Looking For:
Doctors should be well-rounded individuals and should also possess insight. Interviewers want to now that candidates are well-rounded and can work well with others

Example Answer

"My school friends would say that I am intelligent, sensible and calm. Friends at my rugby club would say that I am a good team player and hopefully all of them say that I can also have fun. These attributes make me suited to a career in medicine as being a doctor requires intelligence, team work and an ability to remain calm and enjoy your work"

Although this question may seem slightly unusual it is a great opportunity to demonstrate a number of your qualities.

DO YOU WORK BETTER ALONE OR AS PART OF A TEAM?

Interviewers are looking for appreciation of the difficulties and usefulness of working in teams compared to working alone. Your answer should state that you are able to work effectively in either a team or as an individual. In medical school you will be required to be self-motivated and revise by yourself but will also need to work on group tasks.

Use examples of times you have worked alone and as part of a team and use the below summaries to reflect on the benefits of each.

Individual	Voluntary Work Experience
• Able to be your own boss • Work to your own deadlines • Aware of all parts of a project • Minimises errors in communication • No management of team members is required	• Work can be divided and reduced for each individual • Collaboration and team spirit can make the project more enjoyable • Opinions and views of team members can improve the final product • Improves communication and team work skills • Team members with different skills can be utilised

WHO IS YOUR ROLE MODEL AND WHY?

Interviewers will want to get to know what you are like as a person and what you perceive to be important characteristics. Select characteristics that are useful to a career in medicine.

Select a role model. This can be a family member, teacher or public figure. If you select a public figure make sure you choose someone appropriate and not a D-List celebrity!

Use the **STAR** framework to explain why they are your role model, what they did and what characteristic they have taught you that you may employ as a doctor.

Role Model Characteristics
★ Hard-working
★ Kind
★ Optimistic
★ Decisive
★ Confident
★ Inspirational
★ Enthusiastic
★ Friendly
★ Dedicated

Make sure you use a personal example to demonstrate these characteristics and explain why you found the person inspiring and how you will take this forward as a doctor.

CAN YOU STUDY INDEPENDENTLY?

Medical school requires independent study and it is important that you can demonstrate this. This question may seem difficult to answer. The best approach is to use examples of times when you have worked effectively in your own time to complete a project or revise for an exam.

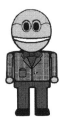

Interviewers Are Looking For:

Example of previous independent study and insight into what will be required at medical school. Revision from books in library, small group teaching, self-assessment and motivation.

Although the question refers to independence remember that you can still study with peers and in small groups to learn topics and practise examination skills.

Attributes to Independence	Study Skills
• Time management	• Text books
• Organisation and setting goals	• Online question banks
	• Practical videos
• Planning work/creating a revision timetable	• Online presentations
	• Mind maps
• Studying with peers	• Short notes
• Self-assessment to ensure you are learning effectively	

Use the **STAR** framework to give specific examples of when you have studied independently.

Example Answer

"As a graduate applicant I was required to attain a high grade in the GAMSAT examination prior to applying to medical school. At the time I was working a full time job and needed to study in my own time to pass the exam.

I first made sure I knew what the format of the exam was and created a revision timetable leading up to the exam covering all topics. I set my revision sessions around my work commitments and stuck to the timetable even when tired at the end of my job. I utilised online question banks and textbooks to test myself and ensure progression in my learning of topics. I also practised with a colleague and spoke with applicants from previous years to get an understanding of what I needed to improve prior to the exam.

I achieved a high score on the GAMSAT and I will take these preparation techniques forward to medical school when revising for end of unit exams."

TELL ME ABOUT AN INTERESTING CASE OR PATIENT YOU SAW DURING WORK EXPERIENCE

Interviewers want to know that you have reflected on your work experience placements and have read around topics discussed. Hopefully you made some notes during your work experience or can recall an interesting case or patient.

Choose a case that genuinely interested you. The condition does not need to be unusual but you need to be able to say why you found the case interesting.

It might be that you empathised with the patient, the doctors may have found managing the patient difficult, you may have seen the patient when they first attended hospital and then when they were treated and went home.

Make sure you say that you were interested and were then motivated to go home and research the patient's condition. Be enthusiastic in your response and ensure you have read around the topic in case you get asked any specifics about the patient, condition or treatment.

Example Answer

"During my orthopaedic work experience placement I saw a 22 year old man who had fallen from a ladder and had sustained an open fracture of his left ankle. As there was an open wound he was given antibiotics and a tetanus booster and had a wound wash out and application of an external fixator in theatre. He was then discussed with the plastic surgeons at a local centre for definitive skin coverage of the wound.

I found this interesting as it showed the multidisciplinary approach helping this patient and the fact that not all services are located on the same hospital site. I also empathised with the patient as he was of a similar age to me.

That evening I went home and downloaded the British Orthopaedic Association and Plastic Surgery Association (BOA/BAPRAS) guidelines on the management of open fractures which highlighted how national guidelines can help to improve patient care."

HOW DOES THE WORK OF DOCTORS AT DIFFERENT STAGES OF TRAINING DIFFER?

This question looks at whether you appreciate how your responsibilities and work change as you progress in your postgraduate training. Use specific examples from your work experience. State what specialty you are using in your example. Describe the roles of Foundation doctors, core trainees, registrars and consultants.

Example Answer

"During my general surgery attachment I shadowed a variety of doctors at various stages of their training.

The F1/2 doctors were mainly ward based. Their day began with a ward round led by the consultant or registrar during which they marked jobs on their list of patients. These jobs included taking blood, requesting scans, reviewing unwell patients, prescribing medications and completing discharge summaries. They then replied to bleeps from nursing staff, attended teaching and raised any concerns to their seniors.

The core trainees also helped with this but also had time allocated to assist in theatre and learn in clinic.

Registrars had more responsibility with their own clinics and theatre lists and liaised with their consultants performing some operations and assisting in more complex procedures.

Consultants led ward rounds, ran clinics and also attended departmental meetings and responded to patient letters and referrals."

FACTUAL QUESTIONS

Interviewers may ask you direct fact-based questions. These are often follow-on questions to push the better candidates or to test your understanding of important medical facts or the course at the medical school to which you are applying. If you don't know an answer it is best to say so and then make an educated guess rather than trying to fluff your way through. Below are a few direct questions that you should know a little about.

What do doctors gain at the end of the F1 year?

Full GMC Registration

What is 'Modernising Medical Careers'?

Modernising Medical Careers (MMC) is a programme for postgraduate medical training introduced in the UK from 2005 onwards. The programme replaced the original 'house officer' grades with the current training structure. It was heavily criticised by Professor Sir John Tooke in his report into medical training.

What is 'Evidence-Based Medicine'?

Doctors use research articles and published evidence to guide their management of patient care.

What is 'Hospital at Night'?

Some specialties such as surgery are less busy at night. To save money and staff the hospital at night programme uses fewer doctors to cover a wider variety of specialties at night rather than lots of doctors with specialist knowledge. The doctor is usually a F1 or F2.

How long does it take to train in medicine/surgery/GP?

Medicine and Surgery around 10 years and GP 3 years.

What is the 'Francis Report'?

The report published by Robert Francis QC in 2013 following his enquiry into failings of care at Mid Staffordshire NHS Trust. The report called for a greater focus on patient care, stronger leadership and corporate responsibility by trusts and openness on failings at trust and departmental levels to maintain patient care.

What is the Health and Social Care Act?

The Health and Social Care Bill was passed in March 2012. The main belief behind the bill is that increasing privatisation will increase competition and the number of organisations bidding for NHS work will lead to better services and drive down prices.

GP commissioning groups rather than the previous primary care trusts (PCTs) will decide how budgets are allocated and how contracts are awarded for hospital services.

The main draw backs to this model are that GPs will be forced to ration resources based on budgets and that GPs may be biased in their allocation of resources. There is also more emphasis on profit and economy of treatments than patient care.

What is the 'EWTD'?

The European Working Time Directive was introduced to 2009 and limits doctors in training to a maximum 48-hour week, averaged over a six month period. It lays down minimum requirements about working hours, rest periods and annual leave. This was to minimise errors due to doctor tiredness.

What is NICE?

The National Institute for Health and Clinical Excellence (NICE) is an independent organisation whose goal it is to set out national guidance for treatments. NICE was created to help reduce the previous 'postcode lottery' where patients in one area might be offered a treatment that patients in another area might not based on funding and allocation of resources in each area as different regions were run by primary care trusts (PCTS) each with different rules and budgets.

NICE analyses current evidence and involves leading doctors in their fields to help develop guidelines and uses QALYs (quality adjusted life years) to decide if treatments should be funded.

Who is responsible for postgraduate training for medicine/surgery/GP?

The respective Royal Colleges dictate postgraduate curriculums for their doctors.

What is 'Gillick Competence'?

Gillick competence is a term is used to decide whether a child (16 years or younger) is able to consent to his or her own medical treatment, without the need for parental permission or knowledge. It may apply to any treatment (compared to Fraser Guidelines which deal exclusively with contraception).

What are extended nurse practitioners?

ENPs or specialist nurses have taken an increasing role in the NHS as the European Working Time Directive has meant that doctors may only spend a limited time working shifts during the working week.

ENPs are nurses experienced in a single field who are able to perform duties previously reserved for junior doctors. Their role may involve taking a simple history, examining a patient or even prescribing drugs. They help to maintain staffing levels and facilitate the roles of doctors rotating through departments.

What do you understand by the term holistic medicine

Holistic medicine or 'whole person care' takes into account not just the presenting symptom but the patient as a whole.

For example a patient with a chronic or terminal illness may be suffering with both the symptoms of the disease together with psychological illnesses such as depression.

Aside from treating patients. What else do doctors do?

Managing patients is at the centre of medicine, however, doctors are involved with many other facets of hospital life and medical education.

Use specific examples from your work experience to guide you.

Roles Of A Doctor
• Teaching students and junior colleagues
• Managerial roles such as rota management, attending departmental meetings
• Quality improvement such as audits and improving patient safety
• Research including writing journal articles and performing lab-based and clinical research
• Writing text books
• Examining and interviewing junior colleagues
• Looking after junior colleagues as a mentor or educational supervisor
• Becoming involved with national committees and improving health care on a larger scale
• Explaining topical issues via the media
• Improving world health by training and helping colleagues abroad

Why is teaching important in medicine?

Doctors are required to teach both medical students and colleagues in order to maintain standards of patient care, improve teamwork and develop their own skills.

What is Problem Based Learning?

PBL is a student-centred method of active learning in which students learn about a subject through the experience of problem solving.

In practical terms students are presented with a patient-centred case and work in groups to devise the most appropriate management options. A tutor acts in a support role to guide the group in their decision-making process and students are encouraged to work together and learn about management options.

What are the pros and cons of Problem Based Learning?

Pros of PBL	Cons of PBL
• Promotes team work	• Does not suit all topics
• Promotes communication skills	• Learning experience dependent on facilitator and team members
• Encourages self-directed learning from an early stage	• Some students may be better suited to lecture-based factual teaching
• Integrates core concepts with practical tasks	• Stark contrast to school teaching
• Requires initiative	• Dependent on quality of cases used
• Evidence shows information is retained for longer when compared to lecture-based teaching	• Best suits students with initiative

Insider Tip

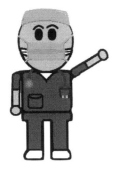

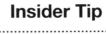

"Interviewers will push the best candidates to see the extent of their knowledge if you get asked lots of specific questions you are probably doing very well."

What are the pros and cons of traditional lecture-based teaching?

Pros of lectures	Cons of lectures
• Students learn basic knowledge before being released on patients	• Does not improve transferrable skills such as team work or communication
• All students receive equal teaching	• Theory only and may not relate to practical application till later in the course
• All topics can be covered equally	• Dependent on the delivery of the speaker
• Students can learn at their own pace	• Students can lose concentration or fall asleep
• Topics presented in a systematic fashion	• Minimal interaction
• Similar to school learning	• Limited or no patient contact

What types of teaching do you know?

- 1 to 1 teaching

    Pros: catered to the individual student, allows gaps in knowledge to be identified and maximizes participation and interaction

    Cons: time consuming, heavily relies on teacher-student rapport, can be intimidating, teaching can be too paternalistic, no learning from peers.

- Small-Group teaching

    Pros: encourages communication and team building, facilitates problem-based learning, teacher acts as mentor guiding group discussion before ideas are shared as small groups come together at the end, students learn from each other.

    Cons: some group members can take over discussion, dependent on participation, requires a set pre-course knowledge level of topic.

- Didactic Lectures

    Pros: Can reach a large audience, can be interactive if pushed

    Cons: not catered to individuals, does not require participation, relies on presenter and slides

- Elearning

    Pros: can reach large number, allow learners to learn in their own time and promotes self-directed learning, allows distance learning

    Cons: needs to be well structured and formally assessed to ensure participation, asking questions can be difficult

What is an audit?

Systematic quality improvement tool comparing current practices with set standards to maintain quality of patient care and outcomes.

What is the audit cycle?

Clinical audit has a number of defined stages. Stages five and re-audit below encompass closure of the audit loop.

- **Stage 1**: Identify the problem or issue

- **Stage 2**: Define criteria & standards

- **Stage 3**: Data collection

- **Stage 4**: Compare performance with criteria and standards

- **Stage 5**: Implementing change

- **Re-audit**: Sustaining Improvements

What is the purpose of an audit?

Goals of Clinical Audit
• Audits are part of clinical governance and are important to patients, hospitals and doctors.
• They maintain standards and outcomes in the healthcare setting.
• They help maintain patient safety.
• They help hospitals identify areas for improvement and help them meet standards.
• They train junior doctors to be analytical and improve their management skills.
• Data collected can be shared with other trusts to implement change on a larger scale.

What is research?

Research is a systematic process to answer a question aiming to create new standards of care and helping to establish best practice.

Research advances medicine and patient care by identifying new knowledge and treatments that benefit patients.

Together with patient care research also helps trusts to improve their reputation and secure funding.

Research helps doctors to develop their understanding of conditions and pathologies, to back up their decisions with evidence based medicine and improves transferrable skills such as analysis, problem-solving and organisation.

What is the difference between research and audit? Is an audit research?

Clinical audit is 'a quality improvement process that seeks to improve patient care and outcomes through systematic review of care against explicit criteria and the implementation of change'.

Research is a one-off, systematic and organised way to find answers to questions. Research does not check whether you are complying with standards, instead its aim is to create new knowledge and new standards.

In essence research helps to establish best practice while audit ensures that best practice is carried out.

What are work based assessments?

Work Based Assessments or WBAs are educational tools used in medical postgraduate training to record competencies and ensure that doctors are meeting targets to progress in their training.

They are recorded using online systems and doctors must have competencies (such as taking blood or examining a patient) scored and signed off by a senior colleague.

At the end of each job placement WBAs are reviewed and any deficiencies can be highlighted to help struggling doctors.

Upon qualifying foundation doctors use the NHS ePortffolio to log their assessments. (https://www.nhseportfolios.org)

What are the differences between general practice and hospital medicine?

Interviewers will want to know that you have done appropriate work experience and have an appreciation for how primary and secondary care differs.

Use specific examples from your time in GP and hospital work experience placements.

General Practice	Hospital Medicine
• General in nature seeing a wide variety of conditions • Community-based • 7 minute consultations at the surgery, phone triage and home visits • Can specialise (GPSI) in certain areas • Training only 3 years in length • Hollistic approach to patient care • Need to decide what can be managed in the community and what needs to be referred to hospital specialists • Need to wait and refer for scans and blood tests • Run as a business with practise managers, GP partners and budgets and targets to meet	• Specialty-specific (neurology, cardiology, ENT, orthopaedics etc) • Hospital-based with theatres, ITU, emergency department, microbiology and pathology services • On call commitments, wards, clinics and theatres • Training is longer 6-8 years after F2 • Instant access to blood tests, scans and referrals

What are the major causes of death in the UK?

• Ischaemic Heart Disease
• Stroke
• Pneumonia
• Lung Cancer

What are risk factors for cardiovascular disease?

Cardiovascular Risk Factors
★ Hypertension
★ Smoking
★ Diabetes
★ High cholesterol
★ Obesity
★ Strong family history

What is the Hippocratic Oath?

The Hippocratic Oath is an oath historically taken by physicians. It is one of the most widely known of Greek medical texts. In its original form, it requires a new physician to swear by a number of healing gods, to uphold specific ethical standards. A modern version is spoken at some medical schools upon graduation.

What is a porcine heart valve?

Tissue Heart Valves are used as replacement heart valves in patients with failing heart valves. They are harvested from pig heart valves (porcine) or cow heart sac (bovine). These tissues are treated and neutralised so that the body will not reject them. Some are mounted on a frame or stent; others are used directly (stentless).

Chapter 4 Ethics

Interview Questions

There are no 'right' or 'wrong' answers for ethical scenarios. Rather interviewers will score you based on your ability to discuss both sides of the argument and demonstrate basic knowledge of the ethical principles pertinent to medicine.

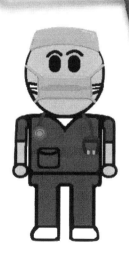

ETHICAL QUESTIONS

e.g. Here is a scenario, there is no right or wrong answer to this. Could you briefly summarise an argument?

Ethical questions cover the ability of candidates to think on their feet and to develop a spontaneous argument. They also test communication skills and candidates' ability to present a rational response. There is often no right or wrong answer and the ability to provide a counter point demonstrates the insight of the candidate regarding the existence of alternative arguments or points of view.

How to Structure an Answer

The '**Four Ethical Pillars**' of biomedical ethics can help you to tackle any ethical dilemma. Remember to read the question, appreciate both sides of the argument and saying that you would involve senior colleagues to help you make a final clinical decision is always a good safety net to end with.

Autonomy From Latin 'auto' meaning self and 'nomos' meaning law. The patient has the right to choose what they want. They may accept or refuse a treatment.

Beneficence From the Latin 'bene' meaning good and 'facere' meaning 'to do'. Doctors must 'do good' and act in the patient's best interests.

Non-Maleficence From the Latin 'male' meaning bad and 'facere' meaning 'to do'. Doctors must not 'do harm' to patients.

Justice Patients must be treated fairly. It mainly refers to the allocation of expensive resources, i.e. it may not be 'just' giving one patient a very expensive treatment if it takes finances away from treatments for other patients.

For any treatment and its side-effects doctors must balance the need to do good versus the potential harm while being wary of resources and ultimately respecting the final decision of the patient.

Other ethical ideas that you may wish to bring in to discussions are capacity and consent.

Mental Capacity The level of understanding that someone has. Some people may have had very limited mental capacity from birth. Other people may develop an illness or suffer an injury later in life that affects their understanding.

Informed Consent Given based upon a clear appreciation and understanding of the facts, implications, and future consequences of an action. Only a patient with capacity may give informed consent.

Common Ethical Dilemmas

There are many potential ethical dilemmas that can be used but by referring to the above principles you can construct a sensible argument for and against each. Common themes are listed below:

• Abortion

• Organ transplant

• Jehovah's Witness blood transfusion

• Animal testing

• Euthanasia

• Sedating a confused patient

ORGAN DONATION: OPT IN OR OPT OUT?

In the UK organ donation is currently 'opt in' meaning that organs can only be donated with the explicit consent of the donor.

Last year in the UK:

- 4,212 organ transplants were carried out, thanks to the generosity of 2,313 donors.

- 1,160 lives were saved in the UK through a heart, lung, liver or combined heart/lungs, liver/kidney or liver/pancreas transplant.

- 3,052 patients' lives were dramatically improved by a kidney or pancreas transplant, 166 of whom received a combined kidney/pancreas transplant.

- A further 3,697 people had their sight restored through a cornea transplant.

- However the UK is still short of donors with recipients waiting long periods for suitable organs.

Opting In System	Opting Out System
• An 'opt in' system is currently in place in the UK. • Changing this would require coordination and finance. • Opt in limits potential donors but respects patients' wishes.	• This would greatly increase the potential pool of donors. • The system would require donors to complete paperwork in order to not donate their organs potentially deterring people from opting out. • The system might not take into account religious beliefs. • The system would require a large amount of finance and coordination to find suitable matches and to ensure organs are not wasted.

SHOULD THE WEALTHY PAY FOR HEALTHCARE?

It is important to note that the question is vague and does not set an income threshold for 'wealthy'. Clearly there will be a large discrepancy in income between patients and those at the lower end of any threshold would be most disadvantaged. There is also no mention of whether this includes emergency care or just elective care.

Arguments Against:
- Everyone should pay the same
- Wealthy people may have worked hard for their money and should not be disadvantaged
- There is already an option for private healthcare
- Some people may be put off attending the doctor leading to more serious complications before first presentation
- Patients may choose the cheapest option over the best
- Patients with chronic illnesses would pay the most
- The doctor-patient relationship would be drastically altered to be based more on money
- Doctors may be biased in advising more expensive treatments
- Patients may turn to alternative therapies or go abroad for cheap alternatives
- May encourage black market healthcare

Arguments For:
- Increase competition between hospitals and practises to drive up quality of care to improve business
- Encourage healthier lifestyles to reduce the need to attend
- Prevent time-wasting patient visits and patients not attending appointments
- Help finance the NHS
- Could reduce National Insurance contributions as payments are made only if healthcare is required

IS IT ETHICAL FOR PRIVATE HEALTHCARE ORGANISATIONS TO OPERATE ALONGSIDE THE NHS?

This issue tackles many of the topics included in the Health and Social Care act. Namely privatisation improving healthcare by driving competition at the expense of creating a tiered healthcare system.

For Privatistaion	Against Privatisation
• The NHS has a limited capacity and an alternative helps to drive down waiting lists meaning that those who do opt for NHS treatment will be seen more quickly if some patients choose to go privately. • Improves competition and services • Offers options that are not offered through the NHS due to budget reasons	• Favours the wealthy and those with private health insurance • Doctors may favour expensive treatments over cheaper options for profit reasons • Not all illnesses benefit from private healthcare, for example trauma and emergencies are best treated at the nearest hospital • Patients may be recommended treatment centres over established doctors by GPs to meet Choose and Book demands

For Privatistaion	Against Privatisation
• Some private healthcare is, in fact, contracted back to NHS departments such as NHS hospitals renting out private wards or offering private scans using their radiology department. • Allows doctors to supplement their income improving job satisfaction • If there was no option some patients may look elsewhere for private care such as going abroad which may not be in their best interests • Private institutions offer patients the option to be seen more quickly, recover in comfort and select their own surgeon.	• Some doctors travel from their normal hospital to work at private centres limiting follow up • Complications from private treatments often fall on the NHS to treat • Is it unethical to not treat patients based on income?

Deliver both sides of the argument and use your own experiences of healthcare from your work experience to offer personal, specific insights.

SHOULD THE NHS BE RUN BY DOCTORS OR POLITICIANS?

Governments and politicians greatly influence healthcare in a number of ways. Although there are often steering groups consisting of doctors the final say on many topics falls within government budgets and agendas.

Both EU and UK politicians dictate a number of core healthcare issues such as:

- Budgets/Funding
- Public Health Initiatives
- Working Hours
- Regulation
- Rationing

Doctors	Against Privatisation
• Have inside, evidence-based knowledge on the best treatments and how patient care could be improved • Take a patient-centred approach • Are intelligent and possess transferrable skills such as team work, communication and leadership that will help them make decisions • Will often favour patients over budgets and finances • Primary goal is medical rather than political	• Look at the county as a whole making decisions within an overall budget • Take a county-centred approach • Removes difficult decisions from doctors

SHOULD PATIENTS BE ALLOWED TO COMPLAIN?

This is a difficult question and requires appreciation of the complaints process. Some patients have valid concerns while others may put in spurious, litigious claims.

Approach:

- Clearly patients should be able to complain if they are not satisfied with any services.

- Most hospitals have a PALS (patient advice and liaison service) that deals with complaints and forwards them to the relevant department.

- Complaints have risen in the past 10 years and this may be in part to the depiction of doctors in the media together with time and financial pressures on doctors.

- Doctors should be protected from spurious complaints that can lead to unnecessary distress.

SHOULD ALTERNATIVE MEDICINES BE MADE AVAILABLE ON THE NHS?

The term alternative medicine/therapies deals with all therapies not recognised by evidence-based traditional medicine taught in medical schools. These include:

- Acupuncture
- Aromatherapy
- Chinese Medicine
- Crystals
- Herbalism
- Homeopathy
- Hypnotism
- Reflexology

The term alternative is important as it suggests patients take these instead of traditional treatments. Complementary therapies are the same as the above but are used in conjunction with traditional therapies.

Against:
- These therapies lack evidence behind their efficacy

- Mechanism of any potential benefits is poorly understood

- Some substances or therapies may be harmful or toxic

- Alternative therapists are not trained doctors

- Therapies are poorly regulated and standardised

- Poorly understood by patients and may deter patients from seeking the most appropriate traditional treatment

For:
- Offers patients choice and confidence

- May confer some benefits though poorly understood

- Many are harmless

- Help promote the spiritual side of medicine and offer the patient support

- An alternative when traditional therapies fail providing the patient with hope

THE EWTD LIMITS THE TIME THAT DOCTORS CAN WORK TO 48 HOURS. SHOULD SURGEONS IGNORE THIS FOR THE SAKE OF THEIR TRAINING?

The European Working Time Directive was introduced in 2009 and limits doctors in training to a maximum 48-hour week, averaged over a six month period. It lays down minimum requirements in relation to working hours, rest periods and annual leave. This was to minimse errors due to doctor tiredness.

Approach:

Surgery is a craft and surgeons used to be trained by doing as many operations as possible under the tutelage of master surgeons.

Due to the limitations imposed by the EWTD today's surgical trainees may struggle to perform enough operations to attain mastery in their field.

This has led to a shift towards competency-based training where more focus is placed on competency rather than numbers of operations performed.

In practise provided surgical trainees are not tired they will often assist with operations in their spare time to gain extra teaching.

SHOULD THE NHS HAVE TO TREAT PATIENTS THAT HAVE SELF-INFLICTED PROBLEMS SUCH AS SELF-HARM OR ALCOHOLISM?

Self-inflicted problems are not just limited to deliberate self-harm or alcoholic other self-inflicted problems may be:

- Respiratory problems due to smoking
- Problems secondary to obesity
- HIV following high-risk behaviour
- Hepatitis and liver cirrhosis following high risk behaviour

- Skin disease due to sun-seeking behaviour

Approach:

It is often difficult to separate out what is truly self-inflicted and what is due to underlying disease or circumstance.

For Treating:

- All patients should receive healthcare
- All transmissible diseases should be treated to help prevent spread
- Many self-inflicted problems are due to underlying psychiatric issues which can be treated

Against Treating:

- Patients may be likely to relapse and not comply with treatments
- Use valuable NHS resources
- Transmissible diseases can be dangerous for doctors
- Treating self-inflicted problems can remove responsibility from the individual and compound their underlying problems

SHOULD THE NHS FUND NON-ESSENTIAL SURGERY SUCH AS PURELY COSMETIC SURGERY?

It is important to understand what the question is asking. Non-essential surgery is an ambiguous term and what is and isn't essential is defined by commissioning groups. Patients can often get around this by arguing their case on an individual basis.

Some non-essential operations might include:

- Removal of a non-malignant lump or bump for cosmetic reasons only
- Laser eye treatment rather than wearing glasses
- Vasectomy rather than using other forms of contraception
- Breast augmentation
- Liposuction

- Bariatric surgery without attempted weight loss
- Hair transplantation

Arguments against funding:

- The NHS budget is tight and offering non-essential procedure would put further strain on this

- Cosmetic procedures often cover psychiatric problems and even following a procedure patients may relapse and want further surgery as a fix for their underlying problem

- All surgery has risks and complications and with the knowledge that the surgery is free patients may be more forward with wanting surgery regardless of risk

Arguments for funding:

- Many patients with minor self-esteem issues may benefit from cosmetic procedures

- Offering these procedures for free will result in less debt for patients who might otherwise seek expensive alternatives

- Trainee surgeons would be greater exposed to these types of procedures

- Not funding may cause patients to seek cheap options that may not be safe or regulated

SHOULD ALL DOCTORS WEAR WHITE COATS AND SUITS?

The 'bare-below the elbows' policy was implemented in the UK 10 years ago to try and reduce transmissible infections. There is little evidence to support this and doctors in the US still wear white coats and suits.

White coats were also thought to act as a barrier between the doctor-patient relationship. Your argument should centre around doctor patient relationship vs infection control.

Infection Control:

- Suits and ties are difficult to clean on a daily basis and convey a risk of passing bugs between patients

- White coats are easier to wash

Doctor-Patient Relationship:

- Patients like their doctors to be smartly dressed however white coats were thought to be a step too far making patients nervous when attending hospital

A 24 YEAR OLD JEHOVAH'S WITNESS HAS BEEN INVOLVED IN A ROAD TRAFFIC ACCIDENT AND REQUIRES A BLOOD TRANSFUSION. WHAT WOULD YOU DO?

Due to their religious beliefs Jehovah's Witnesses prefer not to receive blood products.

The 4 key ethical principles of Autonomy, Beneficence, Non-maleficence and Justice together with capacity are key to answering this question.

Competence/Capacity:

As the patient in unconscious he/she lacks capacity to make a decision about treatment. In emergency circumstances doctors may act in the patient's best interests.

Autonomy:

As the patient is unconscious it is difficult to establish their wishes. It is important to check with family to communicate what is happening and find out if he/she had an advance directive for such circumstances. If the patient does not want a transfusion even in an emergency it is important to respect their wishes.

Beneficence/Non-maleficence

This is an emergency situation and the patient may not have a directive for an emergency setting. If this is the case doctors should act in the patient's best interests and perform a transfusion.

Ultimately if there is any concern a hospital lawyer or ethical lead should be contacted for advice.

WHAT ARE THE ARGUMENTS FOR PEOPLE PAYING FOR HEALTHCARE?

It is important to note that there is also no mention of whether this includes emergency care or just elective care.

Arguments Against:
- Poorer patients will be most disadvantaged
- Denying patients healthcare based on money could be seen as ethically unjust preventing beneficence
- There is already an option for private healthcare
- Some people may be put off attending the doctor leading to more serious complications before first presentation
- Patients may choose the cheapest option over the best
- Patients with chronic illnesses would pay the most
- The doctor-patient relationship would be drastically altered to be based more on money
- Doctors may be biased in advising more expensive treatments
- Patients may turn to alternative therapies or go abroad for cheap alternatives
- May encourage black market healthcare

Arguments For:
- Increase competition between hospitals and practises to drive up quality of care to improve business

- Encourage healthier lifestyles to reduce the need to attend
- Prevent time-wasting patient visits and patients not attending appointments
- Help finance the NHS
- Could reduce National Insurance contributions as payments are made only if healthcare is required

HOW DOES THE GOVERNMENT INFLUENCE PATIENT CARE?

Governments and politicians greatly influence healthcare in a number of ways. Although there are often steering groups consisting of doctors the final say on many topics falls within government budgets and agendas.

Both EU and UK politicians dictate a number of core healthcare issues such as:
- Budgets/Funding
- Public Health Initiatives
- Working Hours
- Regulation
- Rationing

Budgets
The EU and UK governments have an overall budget as outlined by the chancellor. While it is important that money is invested in public healthcare this should not be at the expense of other areas such as education, transport, defines etc.

Public Health
Money can be invested in health campaigns to help raise awareness of illnesses or support vaccination regimes to help save money in the long term. Governments of rely on bodies such as WHO or NICE to help with public health initiatives.

Working Hours

EU regulations restrict doctors to working 48 hour weeks to avoid tiredness. This is controversial and has greatly impacted training and patient care.

Regulation

Government bodies can help to regulate paramedical industries such as the pharmaceutical industry to prevent not efficacious medications being made available to patients outside of seeing a doctor.

Rationing

Difficult decisions need to be made as to which treatments the NHS can provide to avoid expensive, elective treatments.

WHY IS LIFE EXPECTANCY LOWER IN POORER AREAS?

It is important to have a basic appreciation for public health and the difficulties affecting areas of low income. Interviewers want to know that you understand why less money equals a lower life expectancy.

Lifestyle

- Healthy foods and habits tend to be more accessible to the wealthy.

- Habits such as smoking, which is a major risk factor for lung cancer and respiratory problems, are favoured by those with low incomes.

- People with low incomes may not wish to seek medical treatment for fear of losing income due to illness and will only present when their disease is severe.

Lack of Resources

- Health care funding in poor countries may not provide adequate staff or equipment to provide comprehensive health care for the local population.

- Screening programmes to identify early, treatable disease may not be financially viable or practical.

- Vaccination programmes may not be well funded

- Access to health care may be limited due to lack of funding in other areas such as transport or roads

SHOULD DOCTORS TREAT THEIR OWN FRIENDS AND FAMILY?

The current GMC guidance is that doctors should try to avoid treating their friends and families where possible. This can be difficult and interviewers want to know that you can see both sides of the story.

For Treating Friends/Family:
- Can quickly advise them avoiding trips to the local GP
- You may be an expert in the area of their illness and offer the best advice
- You want to help
- They expect you to help and offer advice
- It can be difficult to refuse

Against Treating Friends/Family:
- Difficult if you suggest the wrong option
- Your judgement may be clouded by emotion
- You may know little about the problem
- May cause stress and breakdown of relationships
- Questionable legal standpoint

IS IT ETHICAL FOR PHARMACEUTICAL COMPANIES TO SPONSOR LUNCHES, TRAINING SESSIONS AND CONFERENCES FOR DOCTORS?

Drug companies and device manufacturers are often keen to promote their business by sponsoring the medical events and training sessions. In recent years this has become more regulated so that only educational events may be sponsored.

For Sponsorship:

- NHS has a limited budget and sponsorship helps offers valuable finance

- Doctors have limited perks and lunches and free training helps build morale

- Doctors can keep an unbiased viewpoint and may not be easily influenced by sponsorship

Against Sponsorship:

- Doctors may select drugs or treatments based on sponsorship rather than efficacy

- Research or opinions given by reps for their products often have poor or little research basis

- Industry may pressure doctors to use their products

HOW COULD THE SHORTAGE OF ORGAN DONATIONS BE SOLVED?

In the UK organ donation is currently 'opt in' meaning that organs can only be donated with the explicit consent of the donor.

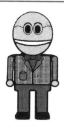

Interviewers Are Looking For:
An appreciation of the ethics behind organ donation together with lateral thinking and problem-solving skills to suggest sensible options to solve the organ shortage dilemma

Approach

There are 2 ways to approach this problem:

1. Increase the number of organs donated

2. Find alternatives to living organ donation with research into better management of diseases or developing alternatives to human organs.

Clearly the second option requires time, money and technology to be viable therefore increasing organ donations is the more immediate solution. It is important to remember that donation relies on altruism and many people may not wish to donate organs for religious reasons. In living patients their autonomy should be respected, the area is blurred when it comes to living donation in brain death.

There are a number of ways to increase the number of donors, each with pros and cons.

Improving the current donation system
At present Spain has the highest number of organ donations in the world and uses an 'opt in' system similar to the UK.

The Spanish system is fairly aggressive with the use of donation co-ordinators who actively seek out suitable donors and talk with their families in the immediate time following death or injury for living donations to discuss possible donation.

While this is effective it is expensive and may be seen as overly aggressive by some as families are most vulnerable in the immediate period following death or brain death.

Changing the system to make everyone a donor
See above organ donation question for more details.

Financial Incentives
Payment for organs is illegal in the UK as it can lead to exploitation and organ trafficking for financial reasons. Poorer countries and individuals would be at risk of selling organs to the highest buyer.

It is also difficult to set a price on organs and who would receive payment. Some more viable options might be discounts for donor card holders or that a set sum is donated to the family estate following death of the donor, however any monetary incentive may be seen to influence a patient's autonomy in making their decision.

Improving Communication and Education

A viable option might be to fund further communication and education on a national/global level regarding organ donation and removing any stigma or anxiety regarding donation of organs. This would require funding and is not guaranteed to succeed.

SHOULD DOCTORS ACCEPT GIFTS FROM PATIENTS?

The bottom line with gifts is that they should not influence a doctor's clinical judgement. Conversely refusing gifts may be seen as rude by patients.

Most doctors accept small gifts. If a patient offers a large gift this is often better directed to the hospital or department to avoid any suggestions of personal gain or bribery. If unsure discussing the gift with colleagues or management is sensible.

For Accepting Gifts:

- Most gifts are meant as a 'thank you'

- Refusing gifts may be seen as rude by patients

- Patients want to show their appreciation

- Most gifts are low in price such as a bottle of wine, chocolates or card

Against Accepting Gifts:

- May be seen as bribery

- Regular gifts from a patient may suggest they are becoming overly familiar

- Large gifts may be seen as taking advantage of patients

- It may seem hypocritical to accept some gifts but not others

SHOULD DOCTORS WHO PROMOTE UNHEALTHY LIFESTYLES SUCH AS OBESITY, ALCOHOLISM OR SMOKING BE DISCIPLINED?

Many doctors smoke, drink or are overweight and this can be seen as hypocrisy by patients if they are being told to cut down.

It is important to appreciate the viewpoint of the patient and of the doctor.

Doctor's Perspective

- Doctors are human too and may find quitting bad habits difficult

- Their unhealthy lifestyle may provide a unique viewpoint that actually helps the patient quit

- Eating, smoking and drinking may help doctors to relax and deal with stress

- Forcing doctors to quit smoking, lose weight or stop drinking is an infringement of their rights

Patients' Perspective

- May lose faith in the doctor as they do not live by their own advice

- See doctors as hypocritical

- May go to see another doctor over a potentially competent doctor due to his/her lifestyle

A 14 YEAR OLD GIRL VISITS HER GP ASKING FOR CONTRACEPTION. WHAT SHOULD THE DOCTOR TELL HER?

In 1985 Mrs Victoria Gillick took her local health authority to The House of Lords as her local GP surgery was prescribing contraceptives to her underage daughters without her knowledge. Mrs Gillick argued that children under 16 lacked capacity to make decisions and GPs were promoting under age sex.

Lord Fraser oversaw the hearing and ruled that a child had competency and autonomy (and that their decision should be respected without informing their parent) if they fully understood the implications of treatment and its risks.

This ruling led to the term Gillick Competence which may be used for consent for all medical procedures and Fraser Guidelines relating exclusively to contraception.

A child is Gillick competent if they are able to understand the risks and benefits of treatment and may consent without their parents' consent.

The Fraser Guidelines are for contraception only and suggest:

- The young person will understand the professional's advice;
- The young person cannot be persuaded to inform their parents;
- The young person is likely to begin, or to continue having, sexual intercourse with or without contraceptive treatment;
- Unless the young person receives contraceptive treatment, their physical or mental health, or both, are likely to suffer;
- The young person's best interests require them to receive contraceptive advice or treatment with or without parental consent.

Approach:
Knowledge of the above is vital as is a balanced view and the ability to assess each patient case by case.

It is the responsibility of the doctor to ensure the child is Gillick Competent and that their autonomy is respected if they are. Conversely doctors must be wary of potential abuse or illegal activity in children asking about contraception.

Doctors should try to persuade children to discuss matters with their parents to avoid conflict.

YOU HAVE ONE LUNG TRANSPLANT AND TWO PATIENTS EACH WITH EQUAL CLINICAL NEED...

THE FIRST IS A 13 YEAR OLD CHILD WITH SEVERE CYSTIC FIBROSIS AND THE SECOND IS A 45 YEAR OLD SMOKER WITH TWO YOUNG CHILDREN. HOW WILL YOU DECIDE WHO GETS THE LUNG TRANSPLANT?

This is a common ethical dilemma with no right or wrong answer. Other variants might include a liver transplant in an alcoholic or cornea transplants in young and old patients. There are a number of factors that you will need to consider.

Begin the scenario by recognising that it is a difficult decision. In reality this decision would not be down to an individual but to a team including transplant co-ordinators and assessors.

Transplant Factors
Although both patients have equal clinical need it is important to ensure both would be suitable for the transplant.

- Are they correctly matched?
- Is the patient fit enough to undergo extensive surgery and recovery?
- Will the patient adhere to immunosuppressive medications to prevent rejection?
- Does either have severe co-morbidities that might reduce life expectancy?

Psychological Factors
- Do the patients want a transplant?
- Will they be able to cope with the immunosuppression regime
- Do they have sufficient support?

- Have they quit any unhealthy habits such as smoking, alcohol, drugs that may impact the transplant?

- Do they have any psychological issues that might cause them to relapse?

Justice

If all other factors are equal you will need to look at what the benefits to society and how best the transplant is used this uses the ethical principle of Justice.

- The younger patient may have more life years to gain in return for the transplant

- The adult has young children who may be impacted by the decision

- The state may need to support the two children costing society more money

- The parents of the child would suffer following her death

- There are no good ways to predict who would benefit society more

Common Assumptions

Be careful to acknowledge but avoid making assumptions about each patient. For example:

- Not all smokers/alcoholics will continue to smoke or relapse damaging the transplanted organ

- The younger patient may not live longer or be of more benefit to society

- The children of the adult may well have other family members and be well looked after

A PATIENT WITH A TERMINAL DISEASE ASKS HIS DOCTOR ABOUT EUTHANASIA. SHOULD EUTHANASIA BE AVAILABLE TO PATIENTS?

Assisted suicide is currently illegal in the UK. The most recent high profile challenge to this was that of Debbie Purdy a multiiple sclerosis sufferer who wanted to travel to the Dignitas clinic in Switzerland to die. She stated that it was within her human rights to do this and would do it while she could still walk rather than involve her husband who may face prosecution for aiding her later in her disease process.

The ethical principles of respecting autonomy and non-maleficence/ beneficence must be carefully weighed up when formulating your argument.

Against:
- Doctors should not harm patients or help them harm themselves
- The doctor must obey the law
- The patient may not be truly competent due to emotion or the disease process
- The patient may not be receiving sufficient psychosocial support

For:
- Some patients may be in extreme pain or distress despite best medical efforts
- Patients with capacity should be allowed to make informed decisions
- Patients' autonomy should be respected

A PATIENT WITH HIV IS REFUSING TO TELL HIS PARTNER. SHOULD DOCTORS BREAK CONFIDENTIALITY TO INFORM PARTNERS IN THIS INSTANCE?

Patients are often reluctant to inform partners about sexually transmitted diseases and sexual health doctors must often weigh up the benefits of respecting a patient's confidentiality and the potentially harmful impact of their partners not knowing they are at risk.

Patient Autonomy

- The patient has capacity and medical ethics state that his/her autonomy should be respected

- Breaking confidentiality may harm the doctor-patient relationship

- The patient may be persuaded to inform their partners if the doctor builds rapport

Informing Partner

- Not tracing sexual contacts and informing partners may cause a large spread of the disease

- If a partner is infected it is the doctors duty to do right by them and in this case beneficence to the partner out weighs the confidentiality of the patient

- Diagnosing HIV and STDs early allows for early treatment and prevention of spread

- A patient knowingly infecting others is illegal and the doctor has a duty to report this

A 15 YEAR OLD GIRL ATTENDS HER GP ASKING ABOUT AN ABORTION. WHAT ARE THE ETHICAL ISSUES?

This is a tricky scenario as it deals with both Gillick competence (is the child able to understand the risk/benefits of an abortion and consent) and also underage sex and possible abuse.

Is an Abortion Viable?
- The first thing to consider is whether the girl is actually pregnant and how far along she is
- If the foetus is >24 weeks abortion is illegal in the UK
- It is also important to try to involve the parents due to potential religious beliefs and the age of the child

Confidentiality & Information Gathering
- The next step is to gather further information about the girl
- How old is the partner?Has she been raped/abused?
- Does she understand what sex and contraception are?
- Is she able to weigh up the implications of an abortion and demonstrate Gillick Competence?
- The doctor should try to involve the parents if possible and if their is a child protection or legal issue inform the police

Psychosocial Issues
- This is a big event for a 15 year old and it is important that the girl has sufficient support
- The parents should be involved if possible
- The GP should build trust with the patient
- The girl should be counselled on pregnancy and STIs
- The girl should be counselled on the psychological effects of terminating a pregnancy and helped to inform her family

A CONSULTANT APPEARS TO BE DRUNK AT THE BEGINNING OF AN OPERATING LIST. WHAT WOULD YOU DO?

Interviewers want to know that you identify this as a patient safety issue but also look for an underlying cause for the consultant's behaviour.

Patient safety

- You will not be on your own so involve senior staff to help you decide what to do

- The main priority is patient safety and removing the consultant calmly from the operating environment

- It is important to report this to the appropriate senior clinician or departmental head as this may have happened before

Supporting a struggling colleague

- It is important to find out why the consultant is drinking

- This might be a one-off mistake due to extreme personal circumstances or may indicate ongoing poor judgement or an alcohol problem

- While it is easy to disregard the consultant's mistake this may be an excellent doctor who needs help

SHOULD TESTING OF MEDICAL TREATMENTS ON ANIMALS BE ALLOWED?

Animals are often used in the testing phase of medications and innovative treatments prior to human testing to ensure safety. Animal activists believe that this causes undue suffering to the animals and is cruel while scientists believe it a necessary step in research. In March 2013 the sale of products tested on animals was made illegal in the EU. It is still acceptable to use rats for experimentation.

For Testing:

- Animals are not humans

- Without animals testing there would be no safe bridge between creation and human testing phase endangering humans

- Dissection of rats and animals following disease helps us to understand about disease physiology and pathology

Against Testing:

- Testing is cruel causing undue pain on animals

- Tests may be carried out a number of times

- Does the advancement of science mean that cruelty is acceptable?

- Animals are defenceless

SHOULD DOCTORS BE ABLE TO GO ON STRIKE?

There is often a dichotomy between the ethical responsibilities of doctors to look after their patients and their ability to protest against government changes to pay, training and factors that directly impact the lives of NHS staff.

In the past 10 years this topic has been discussed when junior doctors free accommodation was removed, when the public sector received a pay freeze and when NHS pensions were re-structured.

Interviewers want to know that you can balance the ethical responsibilities of doctors with the personal right of doctors to protest.

Ethical Responsibilities

Beneficence and non-maleficence dictate that doctors must help and not harm patients. By striking there will be no medical care for patients and this would cause an increase in morbidity and mortality.

In hospitals emergency care would be most affected with patients suffering from serious acute conditions being unable to seek life-saving care. Patients waiting for elective procedures would be inconvenienced and would have to suffer in their current state for longer.

By becoming a doctor and accepting the hippocratic oath doctors have entered into an agreement that they will act in the interests of their patients.

Doctor-Patient Relationship

By striking and showing a disregard for patients the doctor-patient relationship may be irreparably damaged. This could lead to patients being less likely to trust doctors and seek treatment. On a national scale this would add further negative press on the healthcare profession potentially leading to an increase in complaints and litigation.

Autonomy of Doctors

Doctors have the right to protest against changes to their working conditions. The lack of an ability to do so would lead to exploitation of NHS workers, low morale and unhappy staff that may affect the standard of care that patients receive.

Other public sector workers such as police and fire-brigade are allowed to strike.

Striking Alternatives

Cut-Down Service: The way around these issues is to allow doctors to reduce non-essential services. In this way doctors may strike and protest, slowing down the system but not affecting patient care. This might include not completing non-essential paper work or reducing clinics and elective services.

Other Protests: For the removal of junior doctor accommodation doctors pithed tents outside of their hospitals and clearly writing to MPs and creating petitions are alternative ways to highlight work issues.

SHOULD SMOKING BE BANNED?

Interviewers want to know that you can formulate an argument for the health benefits gained to individuals by making smoking illegal and the implications on the autonomy of the population.

For Banning:
- Smoking increases cardiovascular disease, respiratory disease and is a risk factor for lung cancer a major cause of death in the UK
- Inhaling smoke passively can also confer these risks
- Banning smoking would aim to prevent anyone from smoking and inhaling smoke improving health on a large scale

Against Banning:
- Banning smoking removes autonomy from patients
- Smoking may help to reduce stress and a ban may cause patients to seek other ways to relax such as alcohol
- Avid smokers may seek alternatives such as imported cigarettes or marijuana with higher tar or nicotine contents than regular cigarettes.

SHOULD CANNABIS BE DECRIMINALISED?

Cannabis is currently illegal in the UK. It is a popular recreational drug around the world. Cannabis has a number of psychoactive effects including relaxation, introspection, anxiety and paranoia.There is limited evidence for its medical use however in some countries cannabinoids are used to help reduce nausea and improve stress levels in patients with chronic diseases.

Keeping it Illegal
- The side effects of anxiety and paranoia have been linked with serious psychological disease with prolonged use such as schizophrenia
- Cannabis use may lead to harder drugs such as class A drugs such as heroin

- Cannabis sold often contains high tar content and other substances that may cause lung disease

Making it Legal

- Cannabis sold would be standardised removing harmful additives and monitoring tar content
- Already legal in some countries
- May have benefits in chronic disease

IF THE WHO INVESTED £1MILLION IN HEALTHCARE FOR THE DEVELOPING WORLD WHY MIGHT THIS MONEY NOT TRANSLATE DIRECTLY TO THE PATIENTS?

There is a major discrepancy between the quality and access to healthcare in the developing world compared to the rest of the world. The World Health Organisation (WHO) has run a number of campaigns to raise awareness and improve healthcare in developing countries and It is important that doctors are aware of ways they can contribute.

Simply investing money is not a solution as funds may not reach the correct people and areas for a number of reasons.

- Many developing countries have unstable political systems and corruption may not see all of this money spent on healthcare.
- Healthcare includes access to hospitals, staff and resources. The process of building hospitals and training staff takes a considerable amount of time.
- Improving access to clean water, sanitation and vaccinations require planning and co-ordination together with money
- Cultural issues such as the role of women in society may limit the training of female staff and women may be reluctant to get obstetric care

WHAT IS MORE IMPORTANT LENGTH OF LIFE OR QUALITY OF LIFE?

Candidates are expected to formulate an argument for and against each. There is no correct answer and decisions such as this in clinical practise are made based on the specific disease and patient.

Any decision such as this should be specific to the course of disease and the preference of the individual patient. The patient should be given information and support in their decision making process.

- Having a long life allows for more time with friends/family and more experiences

- Life may be prolonged by medical treatments but these treatments may have significant side effects such as nausea, hair loss, pain or tiredness

- Having a good quality of life is important as life is to be enjoyed

SHOULD ABORTION BE ILLEGAL?

Interviewers want to know that you identify this as a patient safety issue but also This is a classic ethical question and has been the centre of pro-life versus choice campaigns for decades. There is no correct answer but interviewers are looking for a balanced argument.

Pro-Life:
- If the foetus is >24 weeks abortion is illegal in the UK, the pro-life argument centres around the fact that there is a grey area surrounding when the foetus is deemed to be alive
- The foetus does not have capacity to decide whether to live or die but should be given the opportunity to be born
- Abortions can be detrimental to the mother conveying both medical and psychological trauma

- Terminating a foetus may be seen as killing an innocent life

Pro-Choice:

- Making abortion illegal removes the mother's autonomy

- Foetuses with chromosomal abnormalities may suffer if they reach birth adding to suffering for mother and child

- Unplanned or unwanted children may have significant financial and psychological implications for the parents and child

- Making abortion illegal may open up women to exploitation by back-street abortion clinics with high-rates of complications

Chapter 5 MMI

Interview Questions

Multiple Mini Interviews (MMIs) involve multiple stations that test qualities of a doctor such as empathy, dexterity, problem-solving, communication and integrity. They may feature traditional and ethical questions together with more interactive and lateral thinking-based assessments.

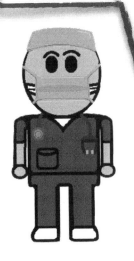

MMI Problem-Solving Tasks

The MMI interview format with its tight time constraints and multiple stations can seem daunting and very different from any other type of interview that you have experienced. The above common questions will feature as individual stations as will extra problem-solving tasks such as the ones below. Each station will focus on a different skill and it is important that you read the brief and focus on what is required.

Explain Your Thinking Process This allows the interviewer to see what you have considered and understand more about how you approach a problem or situation. Try to resist simply leaping to the answer or opinion without explaining how you got there.

Read the Brief In your 2 minutes of thinking outside the room, try to at least come up with some major points that you need to consider in the question.

ONE OF YOUR FRIENDS IS STRUGGLING WITH WORK AT MEDICAL SCHOOL AND OFTEN MISSES TUTORIALS. HOW WOULD YOU TACKLE THIS?

The **SEAS** framework can be used to deal with the problem. The interviewers will be interested in how you tackle this, your empathy and problem-solving skills.

Seek Information

Approach the topic sensitively if your friend is played by an actor start with an open question such as 'how are things?' and let them talk. 'I'm worried about you' is a good phrase for broaching your concerns.

Empathy

Once you know what the reason behind the struggling is try to empathise.

Action

Think about any ways that you can help immediately or offer suggestions to help improve things.

Seek Help

If you feel out of your depth or your friend has a drug or alcohol problem make sure you say that you should involve someone more senior.

AN ACTOR PLAYS THE ROLE OF YOUR FRIEND. YOU ACCIDENTALLY LOST HER DOG WHILE YOU WERE TAKING IT OUT FOR A WALK. YOU HAVE 5 MINUTES TO BREAK THE BAD NEWS TO HER.

This role-play tests insight, integrity communication skills and empathy. You will need to take responsibility for you actions, apologise and show empathy. The interviewers will be marking your tonality, body language and listening skills together with your ability to tackle the scenario.

The hardest thing can be simply stating the bad news. The best thing to do is to give a 'warning shot' such as 'I have some bad news' before telling them straight that you have 'lost the dog'. Give the actor time to react and don't be scared if they become upset. Remember to apologise and empathise with their plight. Do not blame anything else (or the dog) and take full responsibility.

YOU ARE AT THE AIRPORT GOING ON A SKIING HOLIDAY WHEN YOU DISCOVER YOUR BAGS ARE OVER THE WEIGHT LIMIT. PRIORITISE WHICH ITEMS YOU NEED TO TAKE AND WHICH YOU WILL HAVE TO LEAVE.

Skis, Ski Mask, Ski Boots, Hair Dryer, iPad, Ski Jacket, 3 Game of Thrones Novels, Hilarious Ski Hat, Duty-Free Alcohol

Think about how you will prioritise: expense, weight, personal value? It is also worth seeing asking how much over the weight limit you are, whether you can pay for more and whether items could be safely stored at the airport. Be confident and sensible thinking about what you would do in the situation.

YOU ARE LEADING YOUR DUKE OF EDINBURGH SILVER EXPEDITION WHEN YOU NOTICE THAT ONE OF YOUR GROUP IS MISSING. WHAT WOULD YOU DO?

This question is about initiative and resilience and teamwork.

Have a discussion with the rest of the team to discuss what can be done: When was the missing member last seen? How far from the camp site are you? Is there an emergency number?

As leader you must take some responsibility and allocate tasks between all team members. There are many possible options such as sending back a few of the team to check the route, seeking help from a teacher, asking locals or thinking about where he might have gone.

YOU ARE VOLUNTEERING IN A CARE HOME WHEN YOU NOTICE THAT ONE OF THE RESIDENTS HAS NEW BRUISES OVER HER ARMS AND APPEARS MORE FRIGHTENED THAN WHEN YOU LAST SAW HER. WHAT WOULD YOU DO?

This question tests your integrity, empathy and common sense. The **SEAS** framework can be used to help structure your answer.

Seek Information

This is a sensitive issue and you only have very superficial facts with no evidence of wrongdoing by the staff. Gaining more information either from the patient herself, from her family or from the staff is a good start. The patient may have had a fall that has been documented in the notes.

Empathy

The scenario states that the patient is frightened and it is important that you acknowledge this and offer support and see if there is anything that you can do immediately for her.

Action

It is important that the patient is checked for bruising elsewhere as although bruising to the hands may be explained by a fall, bruising on other parts of the body may be more indicative of deliberate harm. Seek help at an early stage and make sure that your findings are documented in the patient notes.

Seek Help

Patient safety is the priority and if there is any concern about harm it is important to highlight this to a senior in the care home at an early stage. If there is any delay or obstruction speaking to someone at school or a doctor may be appropriate.

EXPLAIN TO AN ALIEN HOW TO TIE A KNOT IN A PIECE OF STRING WITHOUT USING YOUR HANDS.

This bizarre example is about breaking down tasks into bite-size chunks and clearly relaying instructions. You might have to clarify that the alien speaks English (and that he has hands!).

Approach
- Fold each end of the lace into a single "loop." You can hold the "loop" in place between your thumb and pointer finger on each hand.
- Cross the loops so that they form an "X" in the air.
- Loop the bottom loop over and through the top loop. This will create a second knot.

- Pull the loops out to the side away from the shoe.
- This will create a square knot that will not easily come undone and will hold the shoe in place.

A CONFUSED, ELDERLY GENTLEMAN IS FOUND WANDERING THE STREET NEAR TO YOUR HOME. WHAT WOULD YOU DO?

This question tests not only your ability to think in a logical manner but also allows you to demonstrate some medical knowledge and empathy. The **SEAS** framework can be used to structure your answer.

Seek Information
Approach the gentleman in a friendly manner and try to ascertain how confused he is. A calm manner will avoid aggravating the confusion. You could use a quick abbreviated mental test (AMT) as is used in hospitals to gauge his confusion. AMT involves asking his name, birthday, age, address, the year, time and date, who the prime minister is and asking him to remember a fact.

Empathy

This gentleman may have a number of underlying problems from dementia to an acute confused state secondary to medication, infection or ischaemic cerebral event. Be patient, do not be flustered and proceed in a calm fashion.

Action

Think about where he might have come from. Is there a nursing home near by or a hospital? Could he be drunk? Provided he is not a danger to you try to get him to sit down and remain calm. See if he has any identifiable information and assess whether he has any injuries.

Seek Help

Do not try to handle this by yourself. Contact the police then any near by medical facilities. Call a friend or relative to help you so that you are not aiding him interlay by yourself.

A FRIEND HAS JUST LOST HIS JOB AND BEEN SUSPENDED FROM HIS UNIVERSITY COURSE. YOU NOTICE THAT HE IS NOT HIMSELF AND IS SPENDING A LOT OF TIME ALONE. HOW WOULD YOU DEAL WITH THIS SITUATION?

The friend may well be experiencing some mental health problems. This could be the causative factor resulting in his job loss such as drug addiction or secondary to this such as a depressive episode. Men in their 20s are at a high risk of depression and suicide and it is important that you ensure he receives adequate support and medical attention.

Seek Information

Fine an appropriate time to talk with your friend and begin with an open question to find out how they perceive things to be going. Think about eye contact, speech and affect as these can give you clues if he is showing signs of depression. Highlight his mood change and see if he has any insight into this or has had any negative or suicidal thoughts.

Empathy

Show understanding about his situation but do not dwell on the negatives. Try to remain positive and formulate a shared action plan.

Action

Ensure that the friend knows that you want to help and that mental health issues are nothing to hide or be ashamed about and that there are people who can help. Arrange to meet again with other friends or plan a social event in the future. Try to get the friend to discuss his problems with a GP who may be able offer further help at managing his mood or just someone outside his peer group to talk to.

Seek Help

Involve your other friends and the friends' relatives if appropriate. The stigmata of mental health issues often prevents people from seeking help and it is important that everyone around the friend knows he needs support.

YOU HAVE AGREED TO VISIT AN ELDERLY LADY AT HER HOME ON A SET DAY. YOU HAVE ALSO AGREED TO ATTEND OF FRIEND'S WEDDING ON THE SAME DAY. HOW WOULD YOU CHOOSE WHICH TO ATTEND? WHAT WOULD YOU TELL YOUR FRIEND/THE LADY?

This is about probity, prioritisation and communication. Interviewers want to know that you can make a difficult decision, be honest and consider ways around the predicament.

- Which did you agree on first?

- Is it possible to change the day you visit the elderly lady?

- What time is the wedding?

If there is no way around cancelling one explain that you would speak to the individual and explain that you will be unable to attend.

Be honest and explain that you forgot about the prior arrangement.

Empathise with the person you are cancelling on and come to an arrangement to meet with them at another time.

HOW WOULD YOU EXPLAIN TO A PATIENT THAT THEY ARE GOING TO DIE?

Be honest with the patient, ensure he/she understands what is happening and show empathy. Do not be afraid to be honest. If there is an actor at the station allow the actor/interviewer time to process the information.

- Introduce yourself

- Show empathy

- Explain that her conduction is terminal and she is deteriorating

- Explain that you need to have a difficult discussion with her about end of life care

- Ask if she would like any family or a nurse present

- Explain what is happening

- Explain that she will be kept comfortable on the ward if she continues to deteriorate

- Give her time to ask questions and show empathy

If this is station is with an actor allow the actor time to digest the information and do not be afraid if they cry. Employ the active listening technique listed in the communication section. If this is simply a discussion with an interviewer

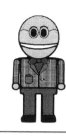

Interviewers Are Looking For:

This question tests integrity and also knowledge of the implications of breaking patient confidentiality.

make sure you use examples you my have seen of doctors breaking bad news to relatives in hospital or while volunteering.

WHILE ON WORK EXPERIENCE YOU LEFT YOUR PATIENT LIST ON THE BED OF A PATIENT. HOW WOULD YOU GO ABOUT ENSURING CONFIDENTIALITY?

This is a common scenario and tests your understanding of the serious implications of accidentally divulging patient information. The priority in this scenario is getting the list back, apologising to the patient, safely despising of the list and highlighting your error to one of the doctors.

Approach

- Introduce yourself to the patient

- Explain what you have done

- Apologise if the patient has read any information

- Explain that you will dispose of the list in a shredder

- Explain that you will highlight your mistake to one of the doctors

YOUR 10 YEAR OLD COUSIN IS VISITING AND WANTS TO KNOW WHAT DNA IS. HOW WOULD YOU EXPLAIN IT TO HIM/HER?

As a doctor you will often need to breakdown medical terms into packets of information that patients and non-medics can understand.

Approach:

- Begin by asking what your cousin already knows. It may be that he/she has a good understanding and this allows you to adjust what you are join to say.

- Use simplistic terms and explain that DNA is complicated

- Explain that DNA is essentially a blueprint for life and is what makes up cells and living creatures

- Explain that DNA is still being studied by scientists

- Use external resources such as the internet to show pictures or links to articles on DNA

A CLOSE FRIEND TELLS YOU THAT HE/SHE HAS BEEN TAKING COCAINE AT WEEKENDS. HOW WOULD YOU RESPOND TO THIS?

This role-play tests your ability to be honest, offer advice and support to your friend. Interviewers want to see you build a rapport, not be judgmental and try to find out why they are using drugs and try to get them some help. If an actor is involved begin with open questions and allow the actor time to speak. Open questions are often employed by doctors to draw out as much information as possible at the start of a consultation before narrowing the questions down and asking about specific things.

Approach:

Ask them open questions such as:

- Are they worried about their habit?

- Are they increasing the amount they take?

- Is everything ok at school/home?

Find out some basic facts first:

- How much are they taking?

- When did this start?

- Why are they taking it?

Do not be judgmental but explain the medical and social implications of taking drugs such as heart problems, psychological problems, anti-social behaviour, addiction and escalation to IV drugs.

Ask if they would like you to involve their family or help them to get help. Do not feel like you need to deal with this entirely by yourself and explain that you think it is important that you involve others for support.

YOU ARE STRANDED ON A DESERT ISLAND WITHOUT ANY FOOD OR WATER. HOW WOULD YOU SURVIVE?

This scenario is about prioritising and using logical reasoning to think about what you would do. Think logically. What would you actually do? What would you prioritise?

Approach:
- Your first priorities are to find food, water and shelter.

- Exploring the island may help you to map out your surroundings, locate food and water sources and ensure that it is actually an island.

- You will not want to expend too much energy in case food/water is scarce

- Building a fire and constructing an SOS sign from rocks may help to increase your visibility to any passing planes or ships

- Is there any natural cover that you can use to make a shelter

- Constructing a receptacle or using large leaves to catch rain water will prevent dehydration

- Keeping hydrated and out of the sun are key

YOUR FRIEND REVEALS TO YOU THAT THEY HAVE NOTICED A LUMP GETTING BIGGER IN THEIR BREAST/TESTICLE. THEY ARE WORRIED ABOUT WHAT THIS MEANS AND ARE SCARED OF GOING TO THE DOCTOR. TALK TO THEM.

This question is about showing empathy and counselling your friend to get help. This is likely to involve talking with an actor.

Approach:
- Begin with an open question to the actor such as 'How are you feeling?'

- Use active listening and do not be afraid to let the actor talk, acknowledging what they say

- Ask them why they are scared. Have they had a relative who has died after a cancer diagnosis or are they afraid of the unknown?

- Encourage them to seek help: if it is nothing serious their mind will be put at ease, if it is more serious they can catch it early.

- Do not be judgmental

- Ask if they have discussed the lump with their parents and encourage them to do so

- Try to finish with a plan but do not worry if the friend remains unsure

YOUR GRANDMOTHER ASKS YOU WHY IS THERE NO VACCINATION FOR THE COMMON COLD. EXPLAIN TO HER WHY THIS IS?

This scenario requires some basic medical knowledge and focusses on explaining the reason in terms that a patient can understand.

While you may want to show off your medical knowledge be careful not to use too much jargon and pitch the explanation at an appropriate level.

Approach:

- Begin by asking what they understand and why they are interested to gauge their level of understanding

- Explain that the common cold is caused by a virus

- There are over 200 varieties of viruses that causes the symptoms of the common cold

- Vaccinations work best when targeted at one specific virus

- As viruses change it is difficult to target all those that cause symptoms of the common cold

- There is however an influenza vaccination of flu jab which is important and has proven to reduce illness in the elderly

YOUR COUSIN IS WRITING AN ESSAY FOR HER BIOLOGY CLASS AND ASKS YOU WHAT CANCER ACTUALLY IS.

This scenario is also about explaining a medical topic in language and bitesize chunks that a member of the public can understand.

While you may want to show off your medical knowledge be careful not to use too much jargon and pitch the explanation at an appropriate level.

Approach:

- Cancer is a condition where cells in a specific part of the body grow and reproduce uncontrollably. The cancerous cells can invade and destroy surrounding healthy tissue, including organs.

- Cancer sometimes begins in one part of the body before spreading to other areas. This process is known as metastasis.

- There are over 200 different types of cancer, each with its own methods of diagnosis and treatment.

- Normal cells can be turned into cancer cells by interruptions and alterations to their normal growth cycle

- These interruptions can be genetic or due to external sources such as radiation or substances known as 'carcinogens' such as cigarette smoke.

- Make sure you check the cousin's understanding and allow them to ask questions.

YOUR UNCLE HAS BEEN TOLD BY HIS GP TO STOP SMOKING. HE DOESN'T UNDERSTAND WHAT GOOD IT WILL DO FOR HIM. EXPLAIN AND ENCOURAGE YOUR UNCLE TO KICK THE HABIT.

This is a common communication skills question and one that GPs have with patients on a regular basis.

Smoking causes cardiovascular disease, lung disease, skin ageing, yellow teeth, fertility problems and is addictive due to it's main constituents of tar, nicotine and carbon monoxide. Passive smoking can also affect family members' health.

Approach:

- Begin with an open question asking about what your uncle understands and what he is concerned about regarding quitting

- Allow him time to speak then try to explain the benefits of quitting

- Explain that quitting is not easy and the average person takes around 5 attempts to stop due to the addictive nature of nicotine

- Explain that the GP can help with nicotine patches and support

- Do not be judgemental, the final decision is your uncle's

Further info:

http://www.patient.co.uk/health/smoking-the-facts

YOUR AUNT JUST HAD A ROUTINE ULTRASOUND SCAN AS SHE IS PREGNANT. SHE ASKS YOU HOW ULTRASOUND WORKS?

This is about explaining a technical procedure to a lay-person. Do not overcomplicate things and use terms that are easy to understand.

Approach:
- Start by asking what your Aunt understands so far.

- Explain that an ultrasound scan, also called a sonogram, is a procedure that uses high frequency sound waves to create an image of part of the inside of the body, such as the womb.

- As sound waves are used rather than radiation, the procedure is safe.

- Ultrasound scans are commonly used during pregnancy to produce images of the baby in the womb.

- Ultrasound scans can also be used to detect heart problems, examine other parts of the body such as the liver, kidneys and abdomen, or help to guide a surgeon performing some types of biopsy.

- Check her understanding and allow her time to ask questions

DURING A MEDICAL SCHOOL MULTIPLE CHOICE EXAM YOU NOTICE TWO STUDENTS PASSING NOTES TO EACH OTHER. THE INVIGILATORS DO NOT SEE THIS HAPPENING. WHAT WOULD YOU DO?

This is a problem-solving exercise and tests your probity. Interviewers want to know that you understand the implications of the students' actions and are able to come to a sensible decision.

Approach:

- You must base your answer on the facts given and not assume anything. The students are passing notes which is a against the rules of most exam settings.

- The implications of this are that they may be cheating and this is a probity issue.

- You yourself are sitting the exam and it is important not to get flustered

- Raising your hand and quietly raising your concern to the invigilator is a good option, this will absolve you of responsibility and allow you to get back to your exam

- The invigilator will then be able to keep a closer eye on the students and will be able to spot any note passing

- If necessary stay back at the end to let the invigilators know

AS A MEDICAL STUDENT YOU ARE GIVEN A SWIPE CARD FOR THE HOSPITAL LIBRARY. A FRIEND WHO IS A LAW STUDENT FINDS THE LAW LIBRARY DIFFICULT TO WORK IN AND ASKS TO BORROW YOUR CARD TO USE THE HOSPITAL LIBRARY. WHAT WOULD YOU DO?

This role-play tests your ability to be honest, offer advice and not be influenced by your friend. Interviewers want to see you stick to your decision, understand the implications and offer alternative suggestions for how your friend can study.

Approach:

- By being given a hospital swipe card you are in a position of responsibility

- Sharing your card with another, non-medical individual may cause trouble for both your friend and yourself

- Although your friend may genuinely want the card to use the library the card might get lost and fall into the wrong hands.

- Explaining that the hospital do not allow you to share the card removes the decision from you and allows you to firmly stick to your decision

- There may be other libraries or places that your friend can go to study which you can discuss with him/her after explaining why they cannot use the hospital library

A PATIENT ATTENDS HIS GP SURGERY FOR A MINOR PROCEDURE TO REMOVE A LUMP FROM HIS ARM UNDER LOCAL ANAESTHETIC. HE IS EXTREMELY NERVOUS. HOW WOULD YOU DEAL WITH THIS?

This is a test of your communication skills. Interviewers want to know you can show empathy towards patients and can also think logically as to how you might alleviate their anxiety.

Approach:
Begin by introducing yourself and building a rapport with the patient. Try to find out why they are anxious; has a friend/relative had a bad experience? have they had a bad experience in the past? Are they unsure of their diagnosis? are they scared of needles or pain? are they confused or vulnerable? do they have a known anxiety problem?

Employ active listening to understand why they are scared and try to answer any questions they may have. Empathise with their anxiety. Explain the process involved that they will be looked after and what the management plan is.

If you struggle to alleviate their anxiety asking their relatives to come in for support or involving nursing staff is a good safety net.

Try to back up your answer with a specific example from your work experience and explain in practical terms how you or the doctors helped an anxious patient.

YOU ARE AT THE AIRPORT WAITING TO FLY WITH A GROUP OF FRIENDS TO SPAIN. ALL OF YOUR FRIENDS ARE IN THE DEPARTURE LOUNGE AND YOU ARE WAITING FOR THE LAST OF YOUR GROUP HENRY TO ARRIVE BEFORE YOU BOTH GO THROUGH SECURITY. HENRY ARRIVES AND REVEALS TO YOU THAT HE IS TERRIFIED OF FLYING. HOW WOULD YOU DEAL WITH THIS?

Interviewers want to know that you appreciate the fact that this is a time-pressured scenario as you are waiting to get onto a plane. Under these conditions you must talk with your friend, show empathy, understand why they are afraid and help them make a decision about whether they want to come on the holiday or not.

The **SEAS** framework may help you to structure the discussion.

Seek Information
Approach the topic sensitively if your friend is played by an actor start with an open question such as 'how are things?' and let them talk.

It may be that they are just anxious or it may be that they have a full-blown phobia and have been unable to get onto a plane in the past.

Empathy
Once you know what the reason behind the anxiety try to empathise and be non-judgemental.

Action
Think about any ways that you can help immediately or offer suggestions to help improve things.

This might include explaining that you have flown many times before and planes are safe or that the whole group will help him/her through it. Ultimately the decision is down to your friend.

Seek Help

- Informing your friends is important to explain the situation. If your friend is too scared to get on the plane it may be that your other friends can offer some suggestions.

- Getting your friend's parents involved is also a way to offer support

- There may also be other ways to get to and from the holiday destination such as by train which may be an option if your friend definitely does not want to fly.

AS YOU ARE LEAVING LECTURES YOU NOTICE THAT ONE OF YOUR FRIENDS IS CRYING. SHE TELLS YOU THAT HER FATHER HAS BEEN UNWELL. TALK WITH HER.

This question is about showing empathy and counselling your friend. Your friend will be played by an actor and your listening, empathy and communication skills will be assessed.

The **SEAS** framework may help you to structure the discussion.

Seek Information

- Approach the topic sensitively if your friend is played by an actor start with an open question such as 'how are things?' and let them talk.

- Find out what is going on and ensure that your friend has support and someone to talk to

- If he/she is very affected enquire whether he/she has informed the university as it may be an option to take some time off studying to be at home

Empathy

- Once you know what the reason behind the crying is try to empathise and offer support

Action

- Think about any ways that you can help immediately or offer suggestions to help improve things.

- This could be as simple as going for a coffee to talk things over

- Arrange a time to meet up again to see how he/she is getting on

- Let them know that they can talk to you at any point if they would like to

Seek Help

- Encourage him/her to speak with family and also the university support services

- Let his/her housemates know that she is upset but let him/her give them specifics

---

RICHARD IS A 22 YEAR-OLD JEHOVAH WITNESS WHO WAS INVOLVED IN A MOTORCYCLE CRASH AND SUSTAINED A PELVIC FRACTURE. HE UNDERWENT SURGERY AND HIS POST-OP HB IS 6.5 (ANYTHING BELOW 8.0 REQUIRES A TRANSFUSION). HE HAS CAPACITY AND IS REFUSING ANY BLOOD PRODUCTS. TALK WITH RICHARD

This is a tricky scenario. Taking the information at face value he has capacity and is an adult so cannot be forced to have treatment against his will. This scenario may well involve an actor.

It is important to make sure that he understands the severity of his low blood count and that is could cause him to have a cardiac arrest if his blood volume drops too low. Find out if there are any family members who could help him make a decision. Explore why he does not want the blood. Don't worry if he still doesn't accept it at the end of the consultation

Approach

- Introduce yourself

- Ask him what he understands has happened and why he needs blood

- Ask him what his concerns are

- Explain the problems if he doesn't have a transfusion (breathlessness, tired, lack of oxygen getting to tissues and at worst hypovolaemia and death)

- Ask if there are any family members he could discuss the matter with

- Explain that you cannot force him to have the transfusion but believe it is in his best interests

- If he asks about alternatives explain that RBCs are the choice product but you will endeavour to find out if there is a local protocol for Jehovah's Witnesses

THERE IS A FIRE ON THE HOSPITAL WARD THAT YOU WORK ON. YOU ARE THE ONLY DOCTOR PRESENT AND THE NURSING STAFF WANT TO KNOW WHICH PATIENTS SHOULD BE EVACUATED FIRST. THE WARD HAS A MIX OF 22 ELECTIVE AND EMERGENCY PATIENTS. HOW WILL YOU DECIDE?

This is about probity, prioritisation and communication. Interviewers want to know that you can make a difficult decision and consider ways around the predicament.

Approach:
- Begin by finding out how many nurses and staff are available on the ward

- It is also important to ensure you know where the meeting point for fires is and that the hospital switchboard have been notified to send help

- It is also important to look at where the fire is and how severe it is.

- The elective patients and trauma patients who are able to mobilise can be helped out quickly to the fire meeting point but should be supervised by at least one member of staff

- Patients that are confined to beds or who are unwell will need 1-2 members of staff to push their beds or transfer them into wheelchairs to help get them out

- Ensuring that connecting fire doors are closed will help stop the fire rom spreading to other wards

- You can either lead by observing from a distance and help co-ordinate the effort or get stuck in and help to get patients out of the ward

YOU ARE GETTING READY TO OBSERVE AN OPERATION. BOTH YOU AND YOUR FRIEND ARE GETTING CHANGED INTO SCRUBS BEFORE GOING IN TO THEATRE. THERE IS ONLY ONE SCRUB TOP REMAINING. HOW WILL YOU DECIDE WHO GETS THE TOP?

This scenario is about prioritising tasks and discussing a problem with a colleague to reach a sensible decision. Communication is key and lateral thinking and thinking about what you would do in real life will help guide your answer.

Approach

- Begin by explaining the situation to your colleague

- Find out what he/she is planning to do in theatre and how important it is to them to be in theatre this morning

- There are a number of ways around this scenario including asking at the theatre reception if there are any extra tops, if there aren't checking your timetable to see if one of your can come back later in the day is also an option

- If your colleague is being particularly difficult allow them to have the top to avoid being unprofessional in the theatre changing room and raise your concerns with your educational supervisor

WHILE TRAVELLING AROUND THAILAND YOU LOSE BOTH YOUR PHONE AND WALLET. WHAT WOULD YOU DO?

This scenario tests your problem solving skills and ability to think in practical terms. It may be that you have been in a similar situation and you should be encouraged to use examples to help you solve the problem.

Approach:

- Begin by assessing whether you might be able to find them

- Where did you last have them? Is there an obvious place you could go back to such as a hotel or bar to ask if anyone has handed them in?

- If you are staying in a hotel or hostel it is sensible to return here and use their phone to call home and your bank and phone company

- Your phone may be trackable online

- If you are travelling with friends they might be able to support you while you find a solution

- If you still have your passport or ID your bank may allow you to take some money out from a local branch

- If all else fails the British Embassy may be able to offer some support

We hope you found the book useful and wish you luck in your medical school interviews.

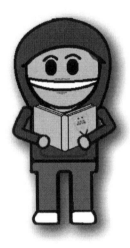

For the latest information be sure to check out

www.getmeintomedicalschool.com

And follow us on Twitter

www.twitter.com/getmeintomed

Printed in Great Britain
by Amazon